Within the Shadow

Scripture teaches that God orders the circumstances of our lives for His glory and for our good. Shelley Chapin's testimony and biblical insights eloquently witness to the reality and the purposefulness of God's discipline. Let her observations bless you as they have me.

—Hudson T. Armerding, Ph.D

Shelley Chapin has confronted suffering and death and found victory in her walk with Jesus Christ and the power of the Holy Spirit. Her teaching and testimony have brought comfort and hope to thousands.

—John W. Neider
Art of Family Living

I highly recommend this book. It effectively addresses an area of life that we will all face one day. It provides both biblical and practical insights for pain, suffering, and death. A must for every church's library.

—Anthony T. Evans, Senior Pastor
Oak Cliff Bible Fellowship
Dallas, Texas

Dealing with suffering and death in the world in which we live is critical for us all. Shelley Chapin gives us some practical and personal insights into how to accept and then grow through the various trials of this life. We believe in what she is doing and recommend this book highly.

—Dr. Frank Minirth and Dr. Paul Meier
Minirth-Meier Clinic

I have known Shelley Chapin for many years, and I know that her life has been enriched by the truths shared in this book. If you are struggling or have ever struggled with any difficulty, then you will relate to and grow from what Shelley has to share with us. All of us need to hear this message.

—Howard Hendricks
Dallas Theological Seminary

WITHIN THE
SHADOW

SHELLEY CHAPIN

VICTOR BOOKS®
A DIVISION OF SCRIPTURE PRESS PUBLICATIONS INC.
USA CANADA ENGLAND

Scripture quotations are from the *Holy
Bible, New International Version,* ©
1973, 1978, 1984, International Bible Society. Used by permission of Zondervan
Bible Publishers.

**Library of Congress Cataloging-in-Pub-
lication Data**

Chapin, Shelley.
    Within the shadow / by Shelley
Chapin.
      p.   cm.
    ISBN 0-89693-186-2
    1. Chapin, Shelley—Health. 2. Me-
sothelioma—Patients—United States—Bi-
ography. 3. Cancer—Religious aspects—
Christianity.
    I. Title.
RC280.L8C48 1991   90-19273
248.8'6—dc20   CIP

1 2 3 4 5 6 7 8 9 10 Printing/
Year 95 94 93 92 91

C o n t e n t s

D e d i c a t i o n

With deepest love and gratitude to:
Mom and Dad,
Knoxie, Bill, Jenna, Barry, and Dorry,
my treasured friends in Tyler and in Dallas,
and to my "other family" — the Hooks.

A special measure of blessing goes to each one who has contributed to the "heart opened wide" in the pages of this book. Without your love and support, I would not know the grace of God in such full measure. As it is, this book represents a tapestry of all our lives, woven together with the unbreakable bond of unity.

Thank you for all that you mean to me. You are loved.

Foreword

There is a great need for the church to have some message of hope and balance for those involved with suffering. Shelley Chapin is a person whom I believe God has raised up to do just that for us all. I have long been impressed by the verse in 2 Corinthians 1:4 that says, "We are able to help those in any trouble, by the same help wherewith we ourselves are helped of God."

I would surely not argue that God sent cancer to Shelley so that she could share this message; but, in a reactive sense, I am grateful that she has given herself to God so that her experience could be of help to those who, for whatever reason, have been unable to hammer out the answers to their personal agonies on the anvil of spiritual experience.

Shelley avoids being morbid while also avoiding sentimentality. This is not easy. Very few people have the poise to walk that fine line and give to us satisfying biblical, personal, and intellectual answers to our questions. She dares then, to offer us spiritual hope that transcends our minds and our emotions. Shelley has helped me greatly with this. In fact, I have thought of myself differently ever since I first became her friend. Although I have no terminal illness, I have come to terms with the fact that only as we all deal with the terminal nature of our existence are we really healthy.

I have found myself on occasion envying Shelley because of the sharpness of her insight into the human condition, her ability to debunk the false values of our culture and to see what really is important and what will last. She does all of this while being a great deal of fun, a delightful friend and companion, intellectually alive and witty—just plain a good person to have as a friend.

This book will give you insights into pain, suffering, and

terminal illness that you have probably not had before. I have read a great deal on this subject and find Shelley Chapin to constantly lead me to new edges of growth. I recommend Shelley Chapin to you without reservation.

JAY KESLER
PRESIDENT, TAYLOR UNIVERSITY

Preface

As this story, my story, unfolds, you will find various passages and insights from Scripture which have been my guides down this newly trodden path of living with pain or difficulty. The verses, stories, and examples in these pages have come to be my companions.

You will also find quotations which have helped me and illustrations I've developed or adopted to help explain the lessons or discoveries I have made. And for those of you who like a challenge, I have included questions at the end of each chapter to encourage you to probe your own understanding of the issues and passages we will consider.

I pray that you will find this book to be much more than a story about one person's experience with suffering. It is a story about how God, in His overwhelming love and wisdom, can take even our greatest fears and deepest pain and work them together for our own good and for the good which He is accomplishing for eternity.

The people I have met, prayed with, wept with, and rejoiced with are all people whom I would not have known in such a way if I had never suffered. The places I have gone and the countless testimonies I have been privileged to give have grown out of God's using what I feared to bring strength and encouragement to me and to others.

The lessons of dependency upon Him and upon family and friends are lessons I would not now trade for any physical well-being. And the pain that has continued to plague my body has actually become a comrade, of sorts, to remind me of all that God has done and continues to do.

This book is about maturity in the hands of God. It is about dying to live and losing to find and trading all that this world has to offer for even a glimpse of knowing Christ Jesus our Lord.

This book is about how to cope and how to help those who are hurting. It is about how to weep and how to share in another person's grief.

This book is about priorities and expectations and yielding control and finding what is really important. In short, this book is about God and my discovery of His love at a level I never knew existed.

1

Life within the Shadow

"This little book reflects my own encounter with the realities of terminal illness and the grief that follows. It is written from the inside of events, not the outside. . . . What I said in the extremes of the agony was as true as I knew how to say it at that time, but I needed to see how well such insight stood up under further living. I am now willing to affirm that the Ground which sustained me then is still firm enough to support the weight of life. I am more convinced than ever that the hope of Biblical religion is authentic vision and realistic perspective."[1]

–John Claypool

A Story That Is Ours

Each of us has a unique story—a story that tells who we are, where we have been, and how God has strengthened and matured us along the way. Our stories are as unique as the mold from which we have been made, and no person's story lacks in significance.

The story told within the pages of this book is my own.

While it is not a complete account of my years, it is the chronicle of an event which has changed my life. Perhaps that sounds dramatic, but it is true.

I came to know Christ at an early age and thought that if I did the right things and made the right choices, I would live somewhat happily ever after. The dream is a common one.

I studied God's Word, was active in church and other evangelical activities, and dreamed of serving God someday. I attended a Bible Church most of my early years and diligently filled notebooks with gleanings of truth.

I had a few dramatic brushes with God along the way, but mostly my walk of faith was a steady one. I spent my summers counseling children at a summer camp—an experience that made a deep impression on my life. I also remember feeling God's closeness in times of real need and sensing the awe of answered prayers. I even heard a few of those sermons that had been written "just for me."

Perhaps the most significant part of my early Christian life was the people who took time to listen to me, love, nurture, and encourage me. Many of these people have since taken their place in my hall of fame, and I will forever be influenced by the care they took with me and my heart.

In short, I had a fairly normal Christian walk—one step at a time, one day at a time. I was well acquainted with disappointments and insecurities, but God had chosen me for His own, and I was on the road to maturity. And then came "the event" of 1982.

Purpose in the Pain

At 28 years of age, I first heard the chilling words that I have cancer. I am one of those people who has enjoyed excellent physical health, and suddenly I was facing the unthinkable. I was not expected to live through the year, but God had something different in mind.

I have continued to live, but not without pain and not without a new way of seeing God and His working in our lives. As followers of Christ, it is my belief that we are strangers here on earth—very purposed strangers amidst the purposed plan of a purposeful, all-loving God.

We try to make this world our home and fit all the pieces neatly in place, but such ease is rarely the guarantee that comes in the package of following Christ. Instead, life is difficult.

Sometimes we must accept pain and suffering and grow in their wake. Sometimes we must yield to God's plan even when it seems to be counterproductive to our own. Sometimes we must step out in faith even when there seems to be no light to guide the way.

When we open ourselves to the workings of the only true God, we must expect the unexpected and trust the One who never relinquishes control. We must let God be God, and discover all that His providence means.

I never knew I would so firmly believe the convictions of my heart, but I do believe in God more than I ever have. I believe in His only Son, our Lord, and in the sufferings that He endured for our sake.

I believe in God's sovereignty in all that occurs in time and eternity. I believe, not only because it is written, but also because I have watched Truth come alive, within and without, over and over again.

The elements of faith I will try to communicate in this book are simple elements, but I think the simple truths bear repeating. All too often we trade them in for more lofty expressions and miss their value in the everyday working out of life.

Although I had studied God's truths and taught them for years, the experiences with cancer and pain have written them on my heart as the very foundations on which life in this world might be lived to the fullest. These elements of faith are the very cornerstones on which I live and breathe and find courage to face each day.

As I begin, let me share with you a few of the premises on which this story is written. Although you will find them in more detail throughout the book, I want to summarize here the lessons that have come to mean so much to me.

I did not understand these premises when I was young, nor did I understand them as well yesterday as I do today. Maturity is a process; coming to know God, an unequalled adventure.

The Gift of Grace

First, it has become more and more evident to me that we live by grace. Our salvation depends on grace, our ability to resist temptation depends on grace, our kindnesses depend on grace, and our days in this world depend on grace.

We act, all too often, as if our days are an allowance which God, as Father, owes to us. We believe that everyone should have a rich and meaningful life, but what we mean by rich and meaningful is often very different from what God means by those words.

In the first weeks and months of my illness, I thought God was robbing me of what was rightfully mine—my life. Even though I knew theologically that I was bought with a price and that I am not my own, the thought of God actually exercising control over my very existence appalled me.

God, You are going too far, I thought.

I was to learn that all of life depends on grace. Each breath I take, every song I sing, every prayer I offer, and every plan I make—all grow out of grace.

Learning to see our lives as a gift, one day at a time, is an important part of living in this world.

The Gift of the Moment

The second premise of my story lies in the concept of time. I have come to realize that the only moment we can be sure about is now. So many times we live for the future, but such living is self-defeating. We will never be any more tomorrow than we begin to be today.

I was stunned by the word *cancer* because I had so many "places to go, people to see, and things to do." Like most of us, I was sure that I would be more fulfilled tomorrow than I am today.

As I faced the illness, I began to see that I will only be more loving tomorrow if I react lovingly today. I will only have more patience tomorrow if I respond with patience at the stoplight or at the meeting or at the grocery store today.

I will only feel more compassionate tomorrow if I look into the crowd and see sheep without a shepherd today. And I will only have enough tomorrow if I look about me with thankfulness and contentment today.

Today is the only day we have for certain to reflect on God's grace and also be reflections of His grace to the world. Today, then, cannot be taken lightly.

The Gift of a Good God

My third premise is the most important of all. Faced with my own vulnerability, I have come to realize that God is completely trustworthy. In a way that I had not needed to trust Him before, I have learned to lay my life, my feelings, my fears, and my needs in the palm of His hand. I can testify that I have found His hand to be loving, warm, and big enough for me.

We say we trust in God, but our trust in Him is tested when unnerving circumstances threaten our security. It is at these times that we wonder if God is really listening, if He really cares, if He is punishing us for some forgotten sin, or if He is just too busy to notice the storm that is threatening to sink our ship.

God is completely trustworthy, and He does not lose His will, His plan, or His people in the midst of the storm.

Central to His very character is the faithful, unchanging quality that causes demons to tremble at the mention of His name.

I think about God's trustworthiness in four descriptions of His nature:

- God is good (Mark 10:18).
- God gives good gifts to His children (Matt. 7:9-11).
- God works, in all things, for the good of those who love Him (Rom. 8:28).
- God intends good, though Satan, this world's ills, and the sin within us may intend evil (Gen. 50:19-21).

If we can grasp that picture, broad and deep and long and high as it is, then we can grasp the breadth of God's sovereignty. Nothing falls outside the realm of God's goodness or His ability to work good—even those circumstances which seem, to us, impossible to bear.

God is good, and He has been at work intending good from before the very beginning of time. Good will be the eternal result of His plan, and good will be the result of His working in each of our lives.

God's goodness is the essence of my faith, my testimony, and whatever strength I possess. The rest of the story is merely the flesh on the all-important skeleton of God's character.

While these truths do not make the circumstances and pains of this world easy, they do give purpose, meaning, and hope to our existence. We are here to give glory to God in all things and to share with a hurting world the comfort and perspective of eternity.

My life "within the shadow" is revealed in the pages which follow. May the experience God has allowed in my life serve to increase your faith and your understanding of how He is working in your life. Our intrinsically good God—the only true God—knows us intimately and has bathed us in His love.

Questions to Consider

1. What are some of your most significant childhood memories?
2. What are some of your most memorable moments with God?
3. When did God become real to you? How? Why?
4. Describe some of the times your faith has been tested.
5. How has God worked good in your life through those times of testing?

2

I Heard the Steeple Chiming

*"A tumor is called benign if its effect is fairly lo-
calized and it stays within the membrane boundaries. But the most traumatizing condition in the
body occurs when disloyal cells defy inhibition.
They multiply without any checks on growth,
spreading rapidly throughout the body, choking
out normal cells. . . . Physicians fear no other
malfunction more deeply: it is called cancer."*[1]
—*Paul Brandt and Philip Yancey*

Once upon a Time

It seems like such a long time since I first heard the word,
cancer. In fact, it seems like the person in the hospital bed
who heard those words wasn't even me. Years have passed,
though not as much in number as in content, and the
illness has taught me more than I can say.

It was late in the summer of 1982, the last week of
August to be exact, when I fell while waterskiing one day.
The fall was not a serious one, but the result was a very
stiff neck that did not want to heal.

As the days passed with no relief, I promised a good

friend that I would go see a doctor about the stiffness. I was annoyed by the inconvenience, but, thanks to God and my insistent friend, I complied.

An Unexpected Guest

"Are you having trouble breathing?" the doctor asked, after examining an X-ray of my chest. I'm sure his face had a sober look as he questioned me, but I took little notice of him at the time.

"No," I replied. "My neck is stiff and I feel tired, but that's all."

He led me into another room where I saw my X-ray, brightly illuminated against an otherwise empty wall. I scanned the picture, but my untrained eyes detected nothing. It looked normal to me: ribs, heart, lungs—the usual.

The doctor pointed out a large shadow in my right chest area, but it made no immediate impression upon me. As I listened to him speak, however, I began to discern that this was some kind of intruder. Saying that he was not qualified to make a diagnosis, the doctor referred me to another physician.

Perhaps any intelligent person would have been nervous at this point, but the reality of any serious problem had not yet found its way into my mind. I had always been very athletic and healthy, so I had no framework through which to process this new information. It almost felt like an adventure—a curious happening.

"Just have a seat, we'll be with you as soon as possible," I heard as I entered a second doctor's office moments later.

The receptionist closed the glass partition and noted the time next to my name on the list. She had spelled my name incorrectly, but that was not unusual.

"It's S-h-e-l-l-*e*-y," I said, under my breath, as I turned. I knew she couldn't hear me, but I thought I might as well set the record straight.

I followed her instructions and found a vacant chair in the waiting area. This office was more colorful and active than the last, and everyone seemed very, very busy.

I was reading a C.S. Lewis book at the time, so I absorbed myself in the story while the nurse tried to squeeze me into the schedule. It seemed like hours before they were ready for me, but it was probably only minutes.

As if he had heard the earlier dialogue, the second doctor asked the identical question: "Are you having difficulty breathing?"

"No," I said again. "But everyone keeps asking me that question. Can you tell me why?"

"There is definitely something growing in your right chest area, but there is no way we can be sure what it is without further tests. I'd like to send you to a surgeon. Do you have anyone in particular that you would like to see?"

I replied that I had a surgeon-friend in Tyler, so, one phone call later I was on my way to the third doctor's office of the day. I now had two X-rays in hand and a growing awareness that something was indeed invading my young and energetic world.

What was next? What would we find? How would this affect my life? The questions rolled over in my mind as I drove, but I had no answers—not yet.

The days that followed held an endless array of tests, needles, machines, and language I had never heard. All of the findings indicated a growing, grapefruit-size mass, but the doctors were evasive with their conclusions.

"It is probably a cyst," I was told. "But there is no way to ascertain the true identity of the mass without surgery."

The date for the operation was set, and I began to prepare for an event that would alter the rest of my life.

The Sober Reality

On October 8, 1982, I was wheeled into the operating room at 6 A.M. I felt groggy from the medication, but I was not too groggy to be soberly aware of my fear. My stomach was tied in knots and so was my faith. For the first time in my life, I felt completely helpless. I could do nothing except wait . . . and trust.

The type of surgery I had is called a thoracotomy. It is a procedure in which the chest wall is opened laterally, from the sternum around to the spine, in order to expose the affected area. I was told it would be a painful procedure, but I did not realize the intensity of the pain I would feel.

I chose to believe, going in to the surgery, that the intruder was a cyst. It seemed unlikely that anything else could be wrong. In retrospect, however, I think that I was just too afraid to consider any alternative.

I remember a friend asking me what I would do if the doctors found something other than what they anticipated. My reply was so naive. "I'll cross that bridge when I come to it," I said, as if discussing the weather for a picnic or some everyday obstacle of life. I just couldn't accept that I might be seriously ill. After all, this sort of thing doesn't happen to someone who is young—and so alive.

When the doctors entered my chest, they found seven malignant tumors, and they had to remove one entire rib and half of another to best protect the area from future intrusion.

Just three hours earlier I had felt so strong; now I was doing battle with a predator I couldn't even see. The prognosis was grim.

"The type of cancer you have is called mesothelioma, Miss Chapin. It is a very rare form of cancer, usually found in older men who have had long-term exposure to asbestos. We expect you will live about nine months."

Those words are a paraphrase of the message I heard from the oncologist. I would tell you exactly what he reported, but I was so shocked and stunned as the words rolled out, that I can only repeat a vague memory.

Nine months? Could I have heard the doctor correctly? Surely he was mistaken! Perhaps my test results had been confused with someone else. I was too young—wasn't I? All I wanted at that moment was for someone to say this was all a dream. I wanted to wake up and find my body intact and my life the same as it had been yesterday. The tears came and stayed—and so did the feeling of helplessness.

Good Company

One of my first comments to a friend seems so simple now, and yet it expresses the nuts-and-bolts thinking of a young person faced with cancer: "Only a few days ago I thought I would live forever. Now I'm going to die."

As I made that simple statement, a light of remembrance turned on in my mind. Someone else had faced that same dilemma, and I had witnessed, in a personal way, the choices he made.

Only six months prior to my illness, I had participated in a seminar on death and dying. A church body in a small east Texas town had suffered many severe losses in a relatively short span of time, and the pastor needed help encouraging his people during this painful period.

The first night of the seminar the speaker introduced the material with the story of a king who lived during the Prophet Isaiah's time. The story was, in many ways, a tragic one, yet it served to teach me a very important lesson.

Hezekiah had been one of the better kings. Coming into leadership at the age of twenty-five, he had battled Israel's idolatry and set a standard for worshiping the only True God. A description of the king reveals his character.

"There was no one like him among all the kings of Judah, either before him or after him. He held fast to the Lord, and did not cease to follow Him" (2 Kings 18:5-6). Hezekiah tried to do what was right in God's eyes.

Then one day, Isaiah the prophet came to Hezekiah, king of Judah, to deliver a message from God: "Get your house in order, because you are going to die; you will not recover" (Isa. 38:1).

Hezekiah's reaction was not surprising—kings are accustomed to dictating plans, not following them. Resembling a child who has just been told no, the king "turned his face to the wall.... and wept bitterly" (Isa. 38:2-3). He had served God faithfully, he felt, and this was no way for God to thank him.

Does that sound familiar? It certainly does to me. My first reaction to cancer was just like Hezekiah's response to his impending death. I wanted to convince God that He needed me to remain in this world. After all, I was faithfully serving Him and was positively more important to Him alive than I would be dead!

Isaiah came a second time to the king with another message from God. It seemed that Hezekiah's tactics had succeeded.

"I have heard your prayer and seen your tears; I will add fifteen years to your life," said the Lord (Isa. 38:5). And with those words, the course of the king's life was changed forever.

Needless to say, Hezekiah was overjoyed! He offered his praise to God, and a peek into his "diary" gives us an idea of the feelings he had and the plans that he made as a result of the news.

> I cried like a swift or thrush, I moaned like a mourning dove. My eyes grew weak as I looked to the heavens.... But what can I say? He has spoken to me, and He Himself has done this. I will walk humbly all my years because of this anguish of my soul" (Isa. 38:14-15).

Such a promise Hezekiah made to God! And I'm sure that the king meant that promise as he wrote in his journal that day. I can understand Hezekiah's fear, I can empathize with his desire to live, and I can feel his joy as God spared him from immediate death. What saddens me is how he spent those final years.

In the last fifteen years of his life, King Hezekiah fathered a son, Manasseh, who became the worst king Judah ever had. And Hezekiah all but gave the nation of Judah into the hands of the Babylonians. So proud was he of *his* recovery, that he showed the enemy all of *his* treasures and all of *his* armories and all of the things in *his* kingdom. (Isa. 39).

What happened to Hezekiah's words of humility? What happened to the plans for his miracle years?

A House in Order?

I often wonder if Hezekiah realized the opportunity he was given. He had the chance to number his days carefully and to keep his house in order. He knew something about his days that few of us are privileged to know. Yet in Hezekiah's anticipation of doing, he tragically missed the responsibility of being. His new years merely reflected the old patterns as he continued in kingly ways.

What Hezekiah thought important in life was the temporary: his years on the earth, his success, and gaining recognition in the eyes of the nations. He achieved those things, in a strange sort of way; yet he missed the joy of throwing everything away for the sake of knowing and imitating God.

Hezekiah thought that the gift of life itself was the miracle. For Hezekiah, however, the real miracle would have been to walk in true humility all of his days.

I knew, as we studied his story that night, that Hezekiah's life held a lesson I needed to learn.

Down to the Basics

As the meeting came to an end that evening, the speaker concluded the session with a homework assignment for the following week. He asked the audience to think about and respond to some important questions: "If you thought you had only a few months to live, how would your life change? What would you do differently?" I remember adding, in my mind, *Who would I want to be?*

I must confess that as I drove home from the seminar that night, I realized I had some thinking to do. Up to that point in my life, I had never even considered the possibility of my own death.

How *would* I respond if my time were limited? I wasn't sure. What *would* be important to me if I had only a few months to live? That question had never even crossed my mind. Who would I be? Why, I'd only begun to discover my identity.

As I lay in a hospital bed, some six months later, Hezekiah's dilemma was suddenly mine, and I had to have an answer quickly to those important questions of life's significance.

Before October 8, 1982 my future had been secure in my mind. I had a list of plans and events that I thought would yield success and fulfillment, and I had only begun to tackle that list.

I wanted a family and another degree or two so that I could teach. I wanted to write books and travel and speak for conferences. I wanted to offer compassion and mercy to people in need. There were so many things that I wanted to do—but now I had no more time in which to do them.

"Lord," I prayed, "my plans are good plans. After all, I only want to serve You. I'm just starting down the road to my future, yet You're wrenching life itself from my grasp. Isn't this a mistake? It doesn't seem fair."

The Pattern of Doing or the Privilege of Being?

My thinking in the early days of my illness reflected a misconception common to mankind. We tend to think of our significance in terms of what we will accomplish. *When* and *as soon as* become the phrases which frame our plans for satisfaction and our dreams for security.

I had once been certain that I would find significance in the "pot of gold" at the end of the rainbow. Now I was at the rainbow's end, and I had some very important discoveries to make.

I thought, long and hard, about how my life should change and what I would like to accomplish in my few remaining months in this world. Because I remembered Hezekiah's life, I knew, somewhere inside, that significance lies in who we are today, not in what we might accomplish tomorrow.

Although my goals once were numerous, I chose two those first few days in the hospital, to characterize my remaining time in this world.

If I only had a few months to live, I wanted to love God with all my heart and to love other people as God has loved me. These are such simple thoughts, yet so full of meaning. Perhaps Christianity boils down to the simple at such times. The choices seemed clear.

Tearing apart my old map would not be easy. Those plans had been part of my dreams for years, and I couldn't imagine feeling significant without them. Yet the new lessons urged me to reject the compulsion of doing and to champion instead, the cause of being. The number of days soon gave way to the value of days, and for that I was thankful.

God had been preparing me for this event long before I knew of its existence. Through Hezekiah's life, He had enabled me to see that there is purpose and meaning in everything He allows. My cancer is no exception.

Time passed slowly in that hospital bed, but I knew I was being given the chance to put my house in order. The only decision that remained was where to begin.

Thursday morning, October 14, the doctor signed the papers for my release. I was free to leave, but I knew I would never be the same. Just seven days after I'd entered the hospital, I was leaving with a completely different understanding of life.

As I pondered all the events and the emotions, my thoughts were broken by the clear chime of a steeple somewhere in the distance. It played a song familiar to my heart, and I listened to the tune until it became my own.

"I hear the steeple chiming,
'How much time?'
'Til my life ceases rhyming
and God's design,
Written on a scroll,
unfolds so I can see
All that He has planned
for me—"

Questions to Consider

1. Think about those times in your life when pain or disappointment has taken you by surprise. How has it made you feel? How have you responded?
2. What is on your list for tomorrow? What do you think will help you feel more significant or fulfilled?
3. Do you value yourself by what you are able to do?
4. If you thought you had only a few months to live, how would you spend that time? What would be your most difficult adjustment? Why?
5. Identify the times when your relationship with God has been characterized by real dependency and trust. What has made the difference in those times? What do you think a life of faith is all about?

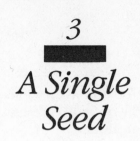

3

A Single Seed

*"Every moment the patches of green grew bigger
and the patches of snow grew smaller. Every moment more and more of the trees shook off their
robes of snow. Soon, wherever you looked, instead of white shapes you saw the dark green of
firs or the prickly branches of bare oaks and
beeches and elms. Then the mist turned from
white to gold and presently cleared away altogether. Shafts of delicious sunlight struck down
onto the forest floor and overhead you could see
a blue sky between the treetops . . . this is
spring."* [1]

–C.S. Lewis

A Long Road Home

Going home in the car after my surgery was an experience
I will never forget. With each slight bump in the road I felt
pain, but I did not care. I was busy gazing at the trees and
the birds and the grass and the sky . . . God's creation had
never looked so beautiful!

A hunger began to grow in me those days that has not

subsided since. I wanted to be as close to the handi-work of God as possible. It soothed me to gaze on His majesty, to touch the creative work of the One who also fashioned me.

On the drive from the hospital that day, I began to see the world through new eyes. I was alive, and my life had new meaning.

Being out of bed and away from the constant care of nurses was a bit of a shock at first. I was unable to get in and out of the shower or go to the bathroom alone, much less dress. The only thing I could do all on my own was sleep, and that did not come easily.

The simplest tasks were no longer simple. It took sheer determination to make the bed in the morning or to brush my hair or to stand from a sitting position. I had never felt so helpless physically or been so deliberate with every move.

I found my lack of ability frustrating at first. If the doctors were correct, I had only nine short months to live. That meant each day passed like sand through an hour-glass, and I was running out of time. I needed my body to cooperate and respond, but I had no way to expedite the process.

Patience became my watchword, and "one more step," my goal. My head believed that God was more interested in me than in what I could accomplish, but my patterns of achievement had been in place for years and would not easily be replaced.

Anyone who has ever been incapacitated for any length of time can attest to the restless impatience of such a situation. The mind can think of a thousand things to do, but it has no legs of its own. I felt the need for activity, but I had no way to satisfy the desire.

I felt small and frail and incapable of having an impact on the world, yet I did know that God was bigger than my frailty. Surely He could use even me—a young, fearful, and unsure cancer patient.

A Journey to Remember

Just seven weeks after my surgery, I was scheduled to make an annual mission trip to Belize, Central America. As you might imagine, no one thought it wise for me to go, but I wanted to take that trip. If I had only months to live, this would be my final opportunity to serve people I had grown to love. I decided to go, and I have never regretted that decision.

Though I had been to Belize several times before, this time I saw the country through different eyes. Everywhere I turned, people just like me were walking around. Their names and faces and circumstances were different, but their needs and fears and longings were the same as mine.

I saw people who need to talk about pain and suffering and death and fear every bit as much as you and I do. And I saw people who believe in a wise and loving God, yet who pray to understand what He is doing and why.

People asked questions about my feelings and fears, and I answered as if I'd known those people all my life. They wept with me in my pain, and I wept with them in the agonies they suffer.

I saw the same insecurities in those people that had plagued me for weeks, and they hungered to hear all that God was teaching me. Suddenly, I had a universe in common with people I once assumed had little in common with my world.

Cancer opened my heart to the people in Belize, and we shared together from a real storehouse of love and grace. The ministry was comforting and real.

I also learned some important lessons about my own significance during that six-day journey. I learned that I do make a difference in this world simply because I am God's child. I learned that He does not need a healthy body but merely a willing spirit to share His Words of Truth.

I learned that my impact on this world isn't measured in the quantity of days that I live but in the quality of love that I give. And I learned that if I am willing to release *my* plans concerning life, God's ways become very clear.

God used my cancer that week to bridge a gap with people who longed for relationships and for understanding. He brought my world right into theirs to show us all how fearfully and wonderfully we are made and how very strong He is in the midst of our weakness.

I was no longer a missionary with a message or a citizen of a country that knows little need, I was a human being—a member of the body of Christ, with a heart. I knew that week that God had big plans for me—a young, fearful, and unsure cancer patient.

A Single Seed

I had prayed, from the beginning of my illness, for some way to feel significant in the months I had left. God graciously granted that request one day in Belize, while sitting on the porch at the home of a missionary friend.

I was reading John 12 about some Greeks who wanted to see Jesus. Andrew and Philip escorted the Greeks to their Master and tried to make introductions, but Jesus would not comply. He had a different plan in mind for the conversation. Instead of making small talk, Jesus responded to His disciples with words that seemed out of place at the time.

> The hour has come for the Son of Man to be glorified. I tell you the truth, unless a kernel of wheat falls to the ground and dies, it remains only a single seed. But if it dies, it produces many seeds. The man who loves his life will lose it, while the man who hates his life in this world will keep it for eternal life (John 12:23-25).

Such strange but glorious words from the Man of Galilee. Perhaps the disciples didn't understand, but I remember feeling a load lift from my shoulders, pound by pound, as I read the passage that day. I had been praying for understanding, and here was God's response. I literally jumped up, turned to my friend, and cried, "This is it. This is the answer to my prayer!"

Not one of the disciples wanted Jesus to die. In fact, when they heard those words, they basically just ignored Him. They were quite determined to keep Jesus alive, and I can understand why.

Jesus was a young man in the ministry, and He was amazing. Who else could walk on water, calm a sea, and feed a crowd of over 5,000 with five loaves of bread and two fish? Who else could heal diseases, restore life, and read people's minds? And who else cared about people the way Jesus cared? He always knew just what to do and what to say in any situation.

He was their teacher, their Lord, their provider, and their friend, and they needed Him to stay. *Let's not talk about death,* they thought, *we've got better things to do!*

Jesus knew a secret, though. He knew that unless the seed is allowed to die, it cannot reproduce. That statement is an obvious one. It describes a reality that we all witness as the death of winter gives way to the vibrant life of spring. We would not argue with the accuracy of Jesus' teaching, nor would we attempt to reject its implications. The application, though—that's another story!

A Single Seed Takes Root

If Jesus had stayed here on earth, the disciples would have rejoiced, but where would we be today? Our burden would now be unbearable.

Because of the suffering and death of our Lord, that "single seed" has produced countless seeds which now proclaim the truth of the Gospel to all the world. Through the sacrifice of our willing Saviour, eternal life is available to all. A single seed for many. That's a deal which now seems to us more than a fair trade.

I began to understand the depth of Jesus' words to Andrew and Philip. I needed to allow God to plant me where He needed me most. I needed to trust the principle of one for many, death for life. I needed, in short, to let go of my plans and let God get on with His.

Each of us has the opportunity to plant seeds of love, grace, forgiveness, and truth as we die to ourselves and live to Christ. Death cannot destroy the kind of seeds He sows through us. We are truth-bearers, and our world needs the life that God has placed within us.

If we hold on tightly to the way we want life to be, we become the losers. One of the most fundamental paradoxes of Christianity lies in the transformation from death to life. For the believer, that which dies begins to live. Jesus knew that principle well.

I had been a Christian for years. I had taught countless Bible Studies and prayed numerous prayers, but I had never quite grasped the concept of dying to myself until I read those words on my friend's porch in November of 1982.

Whether or not God took my physical life, He was asking me to die to my own plans and say yes to His plans. He was asking me to trust Him and to be all that He had designed and awakened me to be.

I became a farmer's hand that day, though definitely a frightened one. I wanted to let God plant seeds through me that would sprout and flourish and grow. Whether people remember my face or not matters little. What I pray they remember is the all-sufficient grace of a wise and loving God who knows exactly what He is doing, even in times of suffering and loss.

The Pain of Growth

> The man who loves his life will lose it, while the man who hates his life in this world will keep it for eternal life. Whoever serves Me must follow

Me; and where I am, My servant also will be. My Father will honor the one who serves Me (John 12:25-26).

Interesting words, aren't they? How do we learn to lose our lives—to hate our lives in this world? The concept seems almost impossible, yet Jesus didn't qualify the words or simplify the command.

The pain of dying to self is very real. I've struggled deeply, as each of you has, with the hurt of suffering and disappointments, of broken dreams and empty tomorrows. Our pain is something God understands, however; He experienced it Himself. That, to me, makes a world of difference.

> He had no beauty or majesty to attract us to Him, nothing in His appearance that we should desire Him. He was despised and rejected by men, a Man of sorrows, and familiar with suffering. Like one from whom men hide their faces He was despised, and we esteemed Him not. Surely He took up our infirmities and carried our sorrows, yet we considered Him stricken by God, smitten by Him, and afflicted (Isa. 53:2-4).

Those words have always haunted me with a firm reminder that Jesus Himself was well acquainted with grief. The God of the universe suffered excruciating pain—the pain of rejection and sorrow, grief and sin.

Had the disciples been given their way, our Lord's suffering and death would never have come to pass. From their limited perspective, such pain was anything but good. Yet what seemed senseless some 2,000 years ago now registers in the heart of the believer as one of the most essential events of history. That which man could not understand at the time has been used by God to give life to death, hope to the hopeless.

There are those who say that Jesus' deity somehow lessened His anguish or invalidated His ability to suffer with us in our agony. I cannot imagine such reasoning to be accurate. Consider which is more difficult—accidentally placing your hand in a fire, or knowingly reaching into that fire to sacrifice a healthy arm for one that is crippled.

Was Isaac's pain greater as he walked up the hill to the altar of sacrifice, or was Abraham the more anguished as he knew what awaited both father and son at the end of the road? Jesus is God, and He clearly knew what was required of Him. Such knowledge did not alleviate the pain; perhaps it even made it worse.

We are told, in the Book of Luke, that Jesus went to the Mount of Olives to pray. Perhaps He wanted an extra measure of grace as He approached the hour of His sacrifice. Perhaps He just wanted the assurance of His Father's presence. Either way, His agony is vivid.

> He withdrew about a stone's throw beyond them, knelt down and prayed, "Father, if You are willing, take this cup from Me; yet not My will, but Yours be done." An angel from heaven appeared to Him and strengthened Him. And being in anguish, He prayed more earnestly, and His sweat was like drops of blood falling to the ground (Luke 22:41-44).

The narrative reveals a Saviour who clearly knew the price He was about to pay—the physical pain of bearing our sin, the emotional rejection of those He loves, and the agonizing burden of feeling forsaken by the Father. And all of this to bring salvation to people who were too self-serving and inconvenienced by His presence to even begin to comprehend the spiritual war that was raging.

When difficult things happen, we want to know why, and we want the solution to come in a bottle or in a counseling session or in a miracle. We fear the unknown—the suffering that seems to have no limit, the loss that seems to have no recovery.

Yet God sees things in a completely different perspective. He is never out of control, asleep, or taken by surprise. He asks nothing of us without cause; He allows no suffering without purpose.

Because Jesus personally suffered, then surely He weeps when we weep and hurts when we are in pain. He is not a Saviour who is distant from our aching, but One who is present and all too aware of what we feel and need. The author of Hebrews brings this truth to our attention.

> Since we have a great High Priest who has gone through the heavens, Jesus the Son of God, let us hold firmly to the faith we profess. For we do not have a High Priest who is unable to sympathize with our weaknesses, but we have one who has been tempted in every way, just as we are—yet was without sin. Let us then approach the throne of grace with confidence, so that we may receive mercy and find grace to help us in our time of need (Heb. 4:14-16).

We are free to approach our Saviour with the longings and fears and needs of our souls. We are free to go to Him and find grace to help us through the painful circumstances of this world. The death of Jesus not only paid for our sins, it also continually provides us with a great High Priest who understands our weaknesses. We are not alone in our pain.

Life is hard, yet the grace to find purpose in suffering is readily available. The only thing we must do is make a choice in the presence of pain—a choice to place ourselves in the Master's care and to see things His way, not merely our own.

"Father, Glorify Your Name"

In the Gospel of John we learn that after searching for food, the disciples returned to the well in Samaria and found Jesus speaking with a Samarian woman. When they urged Jesus to eat, He made a statement that catches my attention every time I read the account: "I have food to eat that you know nothing about. . . . My food . . . is to do the will of Him who sent Me and to finish His work" (John 4:32-34).

The food that was satisfying to Jesus' soul was the food of doing God's will. That's not very nourishing by our standards, but it was completely sufficient for our Lord. He found His satisfaction in doing the will of His Father, even when that included the agony of suffering and death.

In the twelfth chapter of John's Gospel, we read about the choice that Jesus made as He faced the cross, and the simple reason for that choice: "Now My heart is troubled, and what shall I say? 'Father, save Me from this hour?' No, it was for this very reason I came to this hour. Father, glorify Your name!" (John 12:27-28)

In those heartfelt words lies the secret to our living through even the worst of circumstances. God invites the honest expressions of our emotions, yet He longs, at the same time, to be trusted to do what is necessary and good for us.

Jesus told His Father about the pain, and then trusted Himself to the Father's care. He did not lose sight of what He knew to be true about His Father in heaven.

We cannot comprehend God's view of "necessity," nor can we always define His view of what is "good" for us. But we can take comfort in knowing that we are doing the will of the Father. The agony of the events of the Cross could have been nothing short of the deepest anguish, both for Father and Son. And yet, Christ's suffering was mixed with joy. He was doing the will of His Father. Imagine the comfort of such an accomplishment—a comfort available to every believer.

I must say that learning to see life this way is not easy. Each one of us longs to control our lives and, especially, our pain. It is so difficult to trust God when it seems He is, at best, not listening or, at worst, no longer interested in our affairs. Yet He longs to be trusted, just as a father hungers for the trust of his child. To take from God the freedom to do in our lives that which He deems best is to miss the opportunity to see Him work wonders with the very pain we dread. To hold on too tightly to life is to lose that life which we cherish.

The Wonder of It All

I tell you honestly that I have struggled deeply with the thought of dying and with the loss of all that I had once thought life would hold, but I have also learned that God is wiser and bigger and more loving and more aware of my needs and of the needs of His world than I could ever be.

God did not make a mistake in Jesus' life, nor has He made a mistake in the lives of any of His children since the beginning of time. As I look back over the centuries of God's faithfulness, I can only assume that He is no less committed to working out His will in my life as well.

I began to realize, that day on the porch in Belize, that dying to myself gives meaning to my life and to the lives of others. My identity in Christ can never be blotted out by any illness or pain.

"If it dies, it produces many seeds," is an incredible statement of insight and purpose. As we learn to die, we learn to live; and as we learn to trust, we learn to give. The path of dying holds far more living than we can fathom.

That trip to Belize was much more than a last mission trip for me. It was an opportunity to discover a way to live.

Questions to Consider

1. What is the most difficult thing God has ever required of you?
2. What are some plans or dreams or memories to which you need to die?

41

3. What do you need to go to Jesus with right now? What disappointments or experiences do you face now with which you need His help?
4. Think about some of the seed-planting God has done with your life. How has God used you in the lives of other people?
5. What seeds do you think God might be asking you to let Him sow through you today?

4

Through the Eye of a Needle

Silent Night

I would like to report that I came home from the trip to Belize ready to face whatever God had in mind, but that is not the case. I came home with the realization that I *could,* indeed, be a seed planter, but I was still struggling deeply with my fear of the unknown. Turning loose of life itself would not be an easy, one-step operation.

Christmas was drawing near, so all my emotions ran high. If this were to be my final season of family togetherness, warmth, and love, I wanted to experience it all.

"Somebody go outside and check the lights."

"I'll go," I said, as I stepped outside. "It's perfect!" I cried, "Really! Put the star on top, and we're set!"

That bit of conversation has been heard in many a house at Christmastime, yet it marked the beginning of an evening I will never forget.

I was at the home of some friends, helping to "deck the halls" with ornaments they had gathered over the years. We had cut the tree fresh that morning, and it now stood proudly in the corner of the room, displaying its holiday clothes.

Standing on the porch, looking through the window at a room filled with people and laughter, brought back so many memories I had cherished through the years. I also found that it brought an overwhelming feeling of grief. I could not imagine leaving this world or saying good-bye to my family and friends.

"Lord," I prayed, "this is my home. You don't expect me to leave this, do you? Please don't let me die."

I cried long and hard that night. There was so much that I didn't understand about God and His plan for me. I felt lost and alone and very much afraid.

It is a strange feeling to face each day with the knowledge that you are going to die. I felt responsible to make each day count and, at the same time, I felt shackled to a clock that was steadily ticking away the hours of my life.

I have written songs for many years, but the songs stopped coming during those first few months of my illness. I wanted to write, but it seemed as if all I was learning stayed bottled up inside. Afraid of my death, I found myself unable to live.

Christmas of 1982 was painful for me. I wanted the clock to stop ticking away the hours.

The Bookends of Life

Each of us lives between a set of bookends—birth and death. While the bookend of birth is firmly fixed in place, we try to push the bookend of death way into the future. Death is something that happens to somebody else's mother . . . somebody else's child . . . somebody else.

If you've ever moved into a house with built-in bookshelves, you know that one of the first things we do with the space is fill it up with books, trinkets, pictures of the family, and other items of interest. We fill up the space because we are not comfortable with empty shelves. So the items come to rest among the dust on our bookshelves.

If we were to make a list from memory of all the books on our shelves by author, title, and subject matter, we would probably find the task a difficult one. Better yet, if we were to write a paragraph summary of what those books contain, most of us would find the job impossible. Why?

The space on our shelves is filled, not only with what we have read and enjoyed, but also with what we think we might enjoy someday or with what someone else has given us to sample. In other words, the space itself is not of critical importance to us when we imagine that we have plenty.

If the rules changed, however, and we could keep only a certain number of books in our libraries, the selection process would be different. We would look through the items that occupy our sacred territory, and choose only those volumes with significance.

Life is like our bookshelves. We live as if our time is limitless, so we stock the shelves with various tasks, countless activities, and elaborate plans which, in and of themselves, have little meaning. The days become lost in the weeks, the weeks in the months, and the months in the years.

When we think our days are limitless, we tend to "waste the space"—to put off until tomorrow that which we meant to do many yesterdays gone by. Such is rarely the case when a person discovers that the end of life is imminent. As the bookend of death moves in tightly, we see our days differently. Our priorities become clear.

The Rich Young Man

One day, Jesus was approached by a young man who "had it all," so to speak. Not only was he young, but he was also wealthy and successful.

Though there was always a crowd around Jesus, the young man managed to reach the Teacher, and he fell at Jesus' feet. The action of the young man intrigues me. It is not often that we kneel at the feet of another. Our pride gets in the way, and we conquer rather than serve, demand rather than seek.

This searching young man asked Jesus: "Good Teacher . . . what must I do to inherit eternal life?"

Jesus replied: "Why do you call Me good? . . . No one is good—except God alone" (Mark 10:17-18).

Perhaps Jesus asked that question, hoping the man would say, "I called You good because I believe You are God." But the Teacher's question brought no response.

Jesus continued: "You know the commandments: 'Do not murder, do not commit adultery, do not steal, do not give false testimony, do not defraud, honor your father and mother'" (Mark 10:19).

The young man declared: "Teacher . . . all these I have kept since I was a boy" (Mark 10:20).

Mark records that "Jesus looked at [the young man] and loved him," and then continued with the discourse (Mark 10:21). I have lately been touched by that simple description of Jesus' posture. He looked at that young man with love as He contemplated His next move. I can just imagine the gaze that passed between them in that second of silence.

Jesus loved the young man so much that He was willing to sacrifice popularity for Truth—comfort for that which is inherently uncomfortable. There are times when such an exchange is quite painful.

"'One thing you lack,' He said. 'Go, sell everything you have and give to the poor, and you will have treasure in heaven. Then come, follow Me" (Mark 10:21).

Was Jesus' statement a reflection of love? Did He really have to ask the man to forfeit all that he owned? Couldn't He settle on a portion of the whole? A percentage? A promise of future sacrifice?

I suppose the young man remained on his knees, but we cannot be certain of the entire scenario. What we do know is that the young man's face fell as the words left Jesus' lips (Mark 10:22).

Perhaps his eyes had been fixed on Jesus and now he looked away in response to the Teacher's suggestion. Or maybe the young man twisted his signet ring nervously as he considered all that he owned.

Can the good Teacher be serious? Does He know how much wealth is at stake? What advantage could there possibly be in selling all that I own? Is eternal life worth the sacrifice?

I don't know what transpired in those moments of silence, but the young man's mind must have filled with uncertainty, wonder, frustration, and anticipation as he made and re-made his decision. He must have questioned "why" and rehearsed the response over and over again in silence.

Then, instead of rising to obey, the young man rose to disappear. He had counted the cost, and the cost was too high. He had surveyed his earthly investments, and they were far too important to lose.

I imagine that young man found emptiness to be a more haunting and troublesome comrade after that encounter, but we do not know the end to his story. What we do know is that he walked away from the only companion who really matters. He walked away from God.

The Rich Young Man in All of Us

The lesson I was learning that winter, which I didn't understand at the time, was the lesson that Jesus longed to teach this young man: when we hold onto anything more than we hold onto our relationship with God, our priorities are out of line.

The only commandment the young man did not keep was the first one. He had a god all right, but it was not the only True God. His idol was his wealth; the object of his faith, his personal comfort.

The emptiness of serving other gods is clearly illustrated in the story of Elijah and his battle with the prophets of Baal on Mount Carmel. Picture the scene.

Four hundred and fifty misled prophets of Baal placed their sacrifice on the wood. As the contest began, they called to their god to rain down fire and burn up the sacrifice.

> They called on the name of Baal from morning till noon. "O Baal, answer us!" they shouted. But there was no response; no one answered. And they danced around the altar they had made. At noon Elijah began to taunt them. "Shout louder!" he said. "Surely he is a god! Perhaps he is deep in thought, or busy, or traveling. Maybe he is sleeping and must be awakened" (1 Kings 18:26-27).

We could almost laugh at this point, except the story is pitiful. Not only did the prophets believe in a false god, but they also refused to admit their folly. Instead of conceding defeat, they continued their base behavior:

> "They shouted louder and slashed themselves with swords and spears, as was their custom, until their blood flowed. Midday passed, and they continued their frantic prophesying until the time for the evening sacrifice. But there was no response, no one answered, no one paid attention" (1 Kings 18:28-29).

Like the prophets of Baal, we make gods out of our own dreams: the power we think will make us happy, the money we store for security, the possessions we collect to fill up our voids, the health we are sure will satisfy.

My first reaction to being ill was to think, *No! This cannot happen to me! I am too young to die—surely God cannot want my life to end.* And I was not alone in such thinking. I received letters and books filled with cures and promises, and I soon discovered that living is often defined, not by quality of life, but by quantity of time. Very few people, including myself at first, could accept that perhaps God was choosing to work in my life in a way that might even include physical death.

When the rich young man left the feet of our Lord, Jesus turned to His disciples and uttered those words that have become so familiar to us all: "Children, how hard it is to enter the kingdom of God! It is easier for a camel to go through the eye of a needle than for a rich man to enter the kingdom of God" (Mark 10:24-25).

For the man in the story, his riches were god. For the misled prophets of Baal, a man-made image was god. In the months since the discovery of my cancer, physical life had become my god. I was afraid to let it go and to let God's priorities become mine.

The story in Mark could just as easily have been about a powerful man, a beautiful woman, a career-minded lawyer, a health-minded jogger, a determined politician, a convincing preacher, or a talented musician.

Our priorities are no secret. All anyone has to do is examine our lives to see what we count as important. Whatever we are afraid to release—possesses us.

The young man didn't own his riches; his fear of losing those riches owned him. He traded the Giver of the gift for the gift itself, imagining his priorities to be in place.

The Needle's Eye

As recorded in the Gospel of John, Jesus reminded His disciples: "The man who loves his life will lose it, while the man who hates his life in this world will keep it for eternal life" (John 12:25).

Eye-of-the-needle living demands that we turn loose what we hold dear and accept as our priority what God gives. There is no room for all our baggage as we step through the eye of the needle. We are all a bit like the young ruler—we want to become mature in Christ, yet we fear the cost—we hate losing in order to find.

The good news is, I know of no one who's stepped through the eye of the needle and then regretted the decision. When we honor God as God in our lives and seek to please Him, we have peace and security in ample supply.

Consider the words of Solomon: "Now all has been heard; here is the conclusion of the matter: Fear God and keep His commandments, for this is the whole duty of man" (Ecc. 12:13). A fairly forthright statement of priority, I'd say, from one who had it all.

God is more gracious than we can imagine, and He loves nothing more than giving good gifts to His children. What we must grow to understand is God's definition of good gifts.

Jesus knew that if the young man sold all of his possessions, he would not be disappointed. If he had chosen to pass through the eye of the needle, the rich young man would have found purpose, relationship, eternity, significance, strength, compassion, and a whole new way of seeing. Jesus explained it this way:

> I tell you the truth . . . no one who has left home or brothers or sisters or mother or father or children or fields for Me and the Gospel will fail to receive a hundred times as much in this present age (homes, brothers, sisters, mothers, children and fields—and with them, persecutions) and in the age to come, eternal life (Mark 10:29-30).

How I wish the young man had made the choice to sell his belongings.

Through the Eye of a Needle

The bookends of life—birth and death—surround us all. It is not how long we live or what we acquire that makes the space between the bookends valuable. It is, instead, how we live. For whom are we willing to die and for what are we willing to lose in order to find life with Christ? A good businessman has his portfolio in order, and so does a follower of Christ.

I can honestly say that my first step through the eye of the needle was not an easy one, nor was the second, the third, or even the fourth. With each progressive step I have had much to release. What I can tell you is that choosing to walk through the eye of a needle has made all the difference in the world. I still fear, I still struggle, I still long to hold on to the comfortable, but I have learned that releasing my life to God is the only thing that makes sense.

God knows exactly what He is doing, and the benefits of trusting Him cannot be captured in a book. What a privilege it is to learn to live between the bookends—to live a life that will never perish, spoil, or fade. Life on the other side of the eye of the needle is life indeed.

Questions to Consider

1. What would your husband, wife, children, or friends say are your priorities in life?
2. What do you feel are the priorities of your heart?
3. Do you need to make some adjustments in the way you live or in the value you assign to things?
4. Imagine yourself in the place of the rich young ruler. What would you ask of Jesus, and what would He say to you about your gods?
5. What baggage would you have to leave behind in order to walk "through the eye of the needle" today?

5

Hello, World

"Never forget this . . . at any point in life, in a thousand kinds of situations, the answer to the prayer 'use me, Lord, I want to be greatly used of Thee,' can be the hardest thing you have ever faced. It is the answer to this prayer that brings exhaustion of a variety of kinds, and that brings a cost to be paid that almost smashes you and me. There is a cost to being 'used mightily of the Lord,' and there always was."[1]

—Edith Schaeffer

Days of Purpose

January of 1983 proved to be a month of direction from God. A group of ministers, gathered at the Pine Cove Conference Center in Tyler, Texas, asked if I would share with them how it feels to be terminally ill. I was thankful for the invitation. It was a chance for me to help others understand what God had been doing in my life.

I remember the occasion well. My mentor and partner in ministry joined me for the session, and we sat on two stools and spoke of the hurt, the questions, and the fears which had come our way as a result of the illness. We shared the Scriptures that had meant so much in the pain, and I sang some of the songs that best expressed my feelings about my new journey.

Each of the ministers in attendance had something to ask and something to offer, so our conversation lasted long into the afternoon. They too had been jolted by the shock that illness or tragedy can bring into the life of an individual, a family, or a friend.

Before our time was done, most were in tears, and I had standing invitations to tell my story in dozens of churches. I agreed that day to spend what I thought would be my last few months sharing God's grace with others. I had no idea, at that time, what God had in store for me.

Telling others about my journey was a gift from God. The fruit of His work became obvious. I knew He was fulfilling my longing to have Him plant seeds through me as the life I'd been afraid to lose took on new meaning.

The Bookends Widen

The months passed by, and as my nine-month marker approached, I began to realize that I was not going to die on that date unless something very dramatic occurred.

In most situations, when God heals or extends life we rejoice. It is difficult to think of death as a gift, except, perhaps, for those who are suffering tremendously under the weight of an illness.

While I was thankful, in one way, for the privilege of life, in another way I was very disappointed and quite afraid of this new development. You see, I had a whole new situation to ponder and to accept. My battle was far from over.

An Unwanted Intruder

In mid-April of 1983, I began to experience a significant amount of physical pain. At first we thought it was caused by the growing cancer, but tests and X-rays showed the cancer to be under control. The only rationale for the pain was the surgery itself, and for that kind of pain there is no cure. I was faced with an unwanted intruder.

Though the pain was not excruciating, it was present twenty-four hours a day at a level I could not handle alone. Thus began my introduction to pain medication, experimental procedures for pain, and interrupted sleep. My only consolation in those days was the thought of heaven.

I don't know if you've ever tried to explain pain to anyone, but our vocabulary is very inadequate for such an explanation. You can say "it hurts right here" or "the pain is sharp" but you can't express just how that pain feels.

On a scale of one to ten, with ten being the most severe, my pain is always a "six" and, at times, a "seven" or an "eight." Still, that description remains mechanical and tells you very little about what's actually going on in my body or in my mind.

Perhaps you can now understand my mixed reaction to an extended life span. It is difficult to learn to live with physical pain, particularly when the end is not in sight.

I knew I was going to live—at least for awhile. But I also knew I would live with a chronic problem. The pain seemed like an enemy, and I wanted God to remove it from my life. I couldn't sleep, I couldn't find relief and, once again, I found myself feeling helpless and insecure.

Hezekiah was never far from my mind in those days. I thought about his extended life span and, yet, his disappointing finish. He had vowed to be changed by the experience, but he forgot his vow in the thrill of being cured (Isa. 38–39).

Could I live my life differently? What was the key to living in pain and pleasing God at the same time? Where could I turn for an example . . . for encouragement . . . for direction to live my new days?

I knew I had a choice to make. I could either live embittered and angry, waiting to die, or I could live to please the Lord. I could either say, "This isn't fair," or "Hello world, here I am again."

A Frustrated Plan

The end of the Book of Romans gives us a picture of the Apostle Paul's plans for ministry. He had finished the job of sharing Christ "from Jerusalem all the way around to Illyricum," and so he thought it time to go where Christ had never been preached (Rom. 15:19-20). Paul's plan was to visit the church in Rome while en route to Spain. Once in Spain, Paul said he would "preach the Gospel where Christ was not known, so that I would not be building on someone else's foundation" (Rom. 15:20). A worthy pursuit, wouldn't you say?

No one can accuse this apostle of being an undirected man. From the time he met Christ on the road to Damascus until the end of his life in this world, Paul was dedicated to sharing the good news of the Saviour. In fact, I imagine that Paul's contemporaries found him a bit exhausting at times. He rarely put personal pleasure before "business."

Much to his disappointment, Paul's plans for fruitful ministry in Spain fell through. Instead of making another missionary journey, Paul found himself writing to the Philippian church while under house arrest. The apostle whose life was dedicated to the church was now separated from the churches and from his dreams.

Paul could have written a letter demanding his release. In modern-day terms, he might have sued the Roman government or whomever else he thought responsible. Paul could have written letters saying, "Get me out of here! I cannot be used by God unless I go to Spain."

He could have cursed the guards and everyone around him with a bitter attitude. He could even have turned away from God, angry because his Father had failed to protect him from this tragedy.

Instead of complaining about the situation, however, Paul wrote to the Philippians that his pain was not without purpose. In fact, his entire letter is a letter of purpose, encouragement, "dying to self," and the attitude of Christ.

> I want you to know, brothers, that what has happened to me has really served to advance the Gospel. As a result, it has become clear throughout the whole palace guard and to everyone else that I am in chains for Christ. Because of my chains, most of the brothers in the Lord have been encouraged to speak the Word of God more courageously and fearlessly (Phil. 1:12-14).

Aren't those words refreshing? Paul wasn't complaining. He was saying that his unlawful arrest was good! How could he say such a thing? What did he know that the rest of us don't?

The only secret Paul knew was the secret of trusting God. Though his plans had included Spain, God evidently had something different in mind. And Paul was hungry to please God, not to live out his own dreams.

Hello, World

What an example God gave to me in Paul—and the apostle was certainly not alone in his commitment. I began to think of Abraham, Moses, the prophets, Mary and Joseph, Peter, Timothy, John. So many of God's people have had to live with long-term suffering in this world, yet their lives have been a testimony to God's faithfulness. God did not disappoint these men and women or leave them to face the suffering all on their own.

Did Paul's letter to the Philippians hold the answers for my dilemma? Could I too encourage others while in my own "house arrest"?

In his letter Paul opened his heart and grants us insight

into his personal struggle. He wrote of a battle within himself—a battle between his longing to go home and his commitment to stay, and a battle between his fear of the unknown and his courage to face that fear.

> I will continue to rejoice, for I know that through your prayers and the help given by the Spirit of Jesus Christ, what has happened to me will turn out for my deliverance. I eagerly expect and hope that I will in no way be ashamed, but will have sufficient courage so that now as always Christ will be exalted in my body, whether by life or by death. For to me, to live is Christ and to die is gain. If I am to go on living in the body, this will mean fruitful labor for me. Yet what shall I choose? I do not know! I am torn between the two: I desire to depart and be with Christ, which is better by far; but it is more necessary for you that I remain in the body. Convinced of this, I know that I will remain, and I will continue with all of you for your progress and joy in the faith, so that through my being with you again your joy in Christ Jesus will overflow on account of me (Phil. 1:18-26).

Paul had lived a long life of service and frontline activity. The church was well established, his letters were being circulated, and his influence was felt in all of the house churches. Couldn't God take Paul home to be with Him? What more could Paul accomplish? Evidently, much. During the apostle's incarceration, people throughout Caesar's household came to a saving knowledge of God's grace through Jesus Christ (Phil. 1:13; 4:21-22).

For Paul, to live was Christ, even when that living cost him his strength. Paul's life was one of discipline and hard work and single-minded purpose; and he was, I am sure, quite tired. Still, he wanted to serve God rather than serve his own pleasure. "Hello world," was Paul's response to house arrest. He welcomed the situation as one more way to serve the One he loved.

Sufficient Courage

It isn't easy to live with life's demands. Paul well recognized the dilemma. If the apostle were to stay on this earth, he knew he would need courage; in his own power, the burden would be too heavy to bear. And so he petitioned the One who grants courage for just enough to do the job . . . sufficient courage to face the task.

Confronted with house arrest or eternity, the choice, from Paul's perspective, was no choice at all. Yet God needed him to stay. He still had work for Paul to do, and Paul wanted to honor God, no matter what the circumstance.

Though my circumstances differ from Paul's, the Lord spoke to me loudly through this passage. It was fine for me to desire to depart and be with Jesus, but the greater choice was to please God, no matter what He required.

I felt depressed when God did not call me home. I wanted to honor God, but I was frightened. I learned that Paul's message was the one I needed to hear. God wanted me to trust Him with the pain and pray for the courage to honor Him despite circumstances.

My pain has not diminished, but the fear has. I have learned that physical pain can pull us down, but it can also teach us to depend upon the Dependable One—to turn to our Father for the strength that He gives. It is not my problem to plan how I will handle the pain. God has promised to grant me sufficient courage and strength for each day. I have yet to be abandoned.

Watching the Clock

A wise, older friend told me a secret one day. He said, "Never be a clock-watcher."

"A clock-watcher?" I replied. "What do you mean?"

"There is nothing more disturbing to an employer than to walk in at 4:30 P.M. and find the employees already slowing down their pace and packing their belongings to leave. If you are paid to work until 5:00, then you ought to work until 5:00."

"God will call you home when it's time," he continued, "so don't be a clock-watcher." I understood what he meant. It is so much better to go home when it is time but so very important to remain here as long as He needs us, as servants of the Author of life.

Paul's life became a model for me. If he could live with his struggles and still honor God, then so could I. Throughout Caesar's household people heard about Jesus simply because Paul was willing to witness rather than live in bitterness.

I had to say hello to the world again and to the God who will provide exactly what I need to accomplish His will in my life. I had no doubt that the course would be a difficult one, but I also had no doubt that God would be with me as I walked along the path of His choosing.

Questions to Consider

1. Describe some of the ongoing pain you have experienced. What was most difficult?
2. Through your pain, what has God taught you about yourself? About Himself? About others?
3. Is there anything in your life right now that threatens your security? Have your plans been changed or cancelled altogether? What can you learn from Paul about facing fear and disappointment?
4. How does Paul's example during house arrest relate to your life?
5. What about Hezekiah? How do you feel about the choices he made in life? What can you learn about yourself from his story?

6

Welcome Home, Uncle Sam

"Webster defines hope, 'to desire with expectation of fulfillment.' To hope is to anticipate. It is more than dreaming, however. It is possessing within ourselves an expectation that someday there will be the fulfillment of that desire. It will become a reality. Hope always looks to the future, it's always on tiptoes. It keeps us going. It makes a dismal day bearable because it promises a bright tomorrow. Without hope, something inside all of us dies." [1]

–Charles Swindoll

The Truth about Hope

How many times have you heard someone say, "I hope it doesn't rain tomorrow," or "I hope dinner is on time!" I wish I had a nickel for every time I have used the word *hope* to express my desires. The folly of such statements never occurred to me, until I had to rely upon real Hope.

If we live by Webster's definition, then we use the word *hope* rightly to describe the expectation of events we desire to occur. But if we use Scripture's definition of hope, the word means so much more.

Not long after my encounter with cancer, I began to be invited to hospitals and homes to offer comfort to families who were facing tragedy. The order was a tall one.

At first, I found the visits a bit awkward and I felt rather insecure, but after a time I became not only accustomed to the scenario but also comfortable with my role. All people need is understanding, a listening ear, a warm touch, a promise of love, and a message of hope. Unfortunately, I found out quickly how infrequently that message of hope is offered to those who suffer—even from clergy.

What is hope? And what message of hope can we give to the person who is dying? The answer is rather simple, but the realization of that answer takes time—and perspective.

I spent my first Christmas with cancer longing to stay in this world. I couldn't imagine living anywhere else, nor could I imagine giving up all that I had here. Several months into the illness, however, I found myself becoming quite at home with the whole idea of eternity. It was the first time I'd been forced to consider life beyond this world. The more I thought and prayed about heaven, the more my hope took root.

The message of hope, for the believer, is a message of going home. It is not a pipe dream flowing from fear or want. Rather, it is a very real promise flowing from Truth. No believer is ever without hope in this world or the next; it is a gift that can never be wrenched from our grasp.

Home Is Where the Heart Is

Most believers would say without hesitation that this world is not our home. And yet most of us live as if this world is the only home we have.

I believe that grasping the concept of eternity is one of the most important steps in understanding and living a life of faith. Our "now" would not be possible without eternity.

If our lives on this earth have been fairly comfortable and semi-controllable—if we've been content here and able to realize our dreams—then we are probably well rooted in the "home" we have established on earth. In countries less fortunate than the United States, I have heard believers speak of "home" in the same breath as "heaven." But these people are an exception. Most of us choose heaven at the crossroad where this world ends, but we do not see it as home—not yet, not really.

I did not understand my life from the greater perspective because I had always seen this world as my point of reference. It is eternity which serves as the point of reference for the believer, not the here and now. It is the Man of eternity who holds our hearts—even now.

Act 1, Act 2, Act 3

Jesus had just finished a meal with His disciples, when He prepared to wash their feet. John recorded this description of the scene:

> Jesus knew that the Father had put all things under His power, and that He had come from God and was returning to God; so He got up from the meal, took off His outer clothing, and wrapped a towel around His waist. After that, He poured water into a basin and began to wash His disciples' feet, drying them with the towel that was wrapped around Him (John 13:3-5).

The description is important. Jesus was not framing His life or performing His tasks based upon this world's perspective. His life, instead, was framed and motivated by eternity. Jesus knew where He had come from and where He was going, and that knowledge set Him free to live in this world and accomplish all that the Father needed Him to accomplish. This eternal perspective set our Saviour free to serve.

63

I have a notation in the margin of my Bible beside these verses in John: *Act 1, Act 2, Act 3.* Just like a play, yet so much more. Let me see if I can explain.

As I read those verses one day, it struck me that we are all living in Act Two of a three-act play. For many people, Act Two is the only act of which they are aware. They live and breathe and save and purchase and plan and dream for all that they hope to accomplish in this world.

Jesus, however, was keenly aware of the entire play. He was there when the events of Act One took place, and He'll be there for the splendor of Act Three. Such awareness set our Lord free to do His Father's will on this earth.

Eternal knowledge not only permitted Jesus to accomplish the tasks of Act Two with purpose and courage, but it also freed Him to serve those whose knees will one day bend at the mere mention of His name (Phil. 6:10-11). Jesus was secure in His comprehension of eternal significance.

Why should the knowledge of Acts One and Three matter? Anytime we have an understanding of the bigger picture, our ability to live in the here and now is greatly enhanced. One of our toughest battles is fighting insecurity, and an eternal perspective takes care of that battle.

Take a look at the security that surrounds us:

> In the beginning was the Word, and the Word was with God, and the Word was God. He was with God in the beginning. Through Him all things were made; without Him nothing was made that has been made. In Him was life, and that life was the light of men (John 1:1-4).

> Do not let your hearts be troubled. Trust in God; trust also in Me. In My Father's house are many rooms; if it were not so, I would have told you. I am going there to prepare a place for you. And if I go and prepare a place for you, I will come back and take you to be with Me that you also

may be where I am. You know the way to the place where I am going (John 14:1-4).

Though our knowledge is not complete, we too can know, in part, what has been and what will be. When we hold tightly to this world's parameters, we live as if Act Two is the final act of the play. But we are not creations of temporal limit, we have eternal life. What happened in eternity past and what will happen in eternity future have a great bearing upon our lives. When we limit ourselves to this world's time, we lose God's perspective.

Hope That Does Not Disappoint

As Christians, then, we have hope—a hope that cannot be tarnished by this world's events, nor endangered by any act of man or Satan. The very fact of eternity set Jesus free to act, and with Him, the people of faith who have walked upon this earth since time began.

The Book of Hebrews records a description that spans history and hearts. In honoring the men and women of faith, the author wrote these words:

> All these people were still living by faith when they died. They did not receive the things promised; they only saw them and welcomed them from a distance. And they admitted that they were aliens and strangers on earth. People who say such things show that they are looking for a country of their own. If they had been thinking of the country they had left, they would have had opportunity to return. Instead, they were longing for a better country—a heavenly one. Therefore God is not ashamed to be called their God, for He has prepared a city for them (Heb. 11:13-16).

What an incredible testimony! The men and women of

faith pressed on despite this world's pain for the benefit of eternity. Such determination cannot be taken lightly.

Am I willing to do the same? Am I willing to allow God to use me today for His eternal glory? I want the answer to be yes, though I am soberly aware of my limitations.

Perhaps the greatest compliment of all was given to the heroes of faith in Hebrews. God was not ashamed to be called their God. I can see Him walking beside them in the desert, or holding their hands as the lions came to feed, or speaking their names in a whisper as they were sawed in two for their faith. They were headed toward the better country, and God would lead them home. They would not be disappointed.

When Paul wrote to the Roman Church about suffering, he also wrote about hope that does not disappoint.

> Therefore, since we have been justified through faith, we have peace with God through our Lord Jesus Christ, through whom we have gained access by faith into this grace in which we now stand. And we rejoice in the hope of the glory of God. Not only so, but we also rejoice in our sufferings, because we know that suffering produces perseverance; perseverance, character; and character, hope. And hope does not disappoint us, because God has poured out His love into our hearts by the Holy Spirit, whom He has given us (Rom. 5:1-5).

When we speak of hope in the same breath as rain or dinner or even days of life in this world, we miss the bigger picture. We forget so quickly that we were condemned to eternal death because of our sin and that Christ, while we were still sinners, demonstrated His love for us by dying for us (Rom. 5:6-8). Such love is more than we can fathom.

My Hope is built on nothing less

Than Jesus' blood and righteousness.
I dare not trust the sweetest frame,
But wholly lean on Jesus' name.
On Christ the solid rock I stand,
All other ground is sinking sand.
All other ground is sinking sand.[2]

Our hope is eternal, and that hope sets the framework for all that we are and do.

Welcome Home, Uncle Sam

The first Christmas of my illness, I was looking for a country of this world's making. I believed in eternity, but I was not allowing that belief to create the boundaries and the perspective within which I lived. I was afraid of losing this world, almost as if the place Jesus is preparing for me would in some way be "inferior" or not as much "mine."

Thanksgiving Day of 1983 found me a little over one year into my illness and grateful for the growth that God had granted. I spent the day, as usual, with my family in Dallas, as we had a very thankful time together, reflecting on the events of the year gone by.

All the way home, I thought of the ways that God had been working in my life. There had been so many changes, so many marvelous touches of His grace. I marveled, that day, at the ample supply of strength and courage that God had provided. He truly was aware of my needs.

My mom is a worrier, so I am trained in the fine art of calling her as soon as I arrive at my home, safe and sound. On that Thanksgiving Day, she called me first, and there was pain in her voice.

"Uncle Sam is dead," she said. I was stunned. Uncle Sam was my mom's only brother, and he was not an old man.

"What happened?" I asked, trying to think of the best way to offer comfort.

My mom replied that he had eaten a meal of leftover turkey and dressing and then gone to the bedroom to rest. It was there that his heart stopped beating, weary from this world's demands.

I found myself saying how sorry I was for my mom's loss, but I couldn't seem to cry for his death. Uncle Sam was a believer, and somehow I knew he was right where God wanted him to be.

When I put down the receiver, I audibly made a statement that surprised me. With arms held high and a smile on my face, I said, "Welcome home, Uncle Sam." I was overjoyed for my uncle's good fortune.

Only one year earlier at Christmas, I had wept and wept over the horror of leaving my home for eternity. Now, I was welcoming my uncle into that place that is home for all believers. I was envious of his condition, comforted by his peace. The change in perspective had arrived.

Hope was now real to me; eternity, my home. Though I have one foot here in order to serve my God, the other foot is definitely with Him, somewhere in the gardens of heaven.

I had much to rejoice over that Thanksgiving Day. While most of my family members and friends thanked God for the blessing of physical life, I found the miracle to be a spiritual one. What had seemed like a tragedy in my life one year earlier no longer felt that way. I had become thankful for the pain, grateful for the process, and comfortable with my frailty and God's strength.

Just Passing Through

No matter how many messages we hear on hope and eternity, no matter how many times we say we understand, the real comprehension only comes as we allow God to increase our perspective.

When I travel to Eastern Europe, I take one bag, and I pack as little as possible in that bag so as not to weigh myself down with unnecessary burdens. It is a grand feeling, to step off the plane with very few choices in my hand. Everything I need for the journey is right there, and whatever I have left behind is of no use to me.

Sometimes the food is unpleasant or meager. Sometimes the sleeping accommodations are less than satisfactory. Sometimes I contract the local diseases. And often I find that the food or the water does not agree with my body (or vice versa).

Still, for some reason, I find the trips invigorating and when I am home, I cannot wait to return. I feel energized by the teaching opportunities, privileged for the friendships and love, and rested in a way I would not normally experience.

What makes the difference? Why do the very things that cause me to complain at home merely seem part of the day's wages on my missionary journeys?

The difference lies in perspective. When I am traveling, I believe I will go home to my comforts after a few weeks of speaking, so the difficulties don't bother me. I can travel as a stranger and not demand my daily necessities. The experience is temporary, I am merely "passing through."

Seeing ourselves "at home" with the Lord, and merely "passing through" this world as pilgrims with a purpose, is a perspective that will help us tremendously as we live amid our sins, failures, and disappointments. If we hold this world as our home, we are certain to suffer greatly in the aftermath of our frailties.

Fellow Pilgrims

Our fellow believers through the centuries of Christianity have learned and taught others this same secret. They have all had to balance this world's losses with eternal gains, and they have all encouraged their flocks to grasp that which is truly important.

Peter encouraged the scattered believers to live as

"strangers" in this world (1 Peter 2:9-12). Paul told the Philippians that his home was with the Lord and his satisfaction was found in doing the work of his Saviour (Phil. 1:19-26; 3:7-11). We know that Jesus had no place to call His home in this world (Matt. 8:20). And we have all marveled at the simple obedience of the disciples, as they left their fishing nets and other responsibilities to follow the beckoning Christ (Matt. 4:18-20; 9:9).

We seem to be Christians who are living in conflict. We are calling the wrong place home and gaining our significance, power, and purpose from that which is temporary.

Addressed to the Colossian church, Paul wrote a message about death that we all need to read again and again:

> Since, then, you have been raised with Christ, set your hearts on things above, where Christ is seated at the right hand of God. Set your minds on things above, not on earthly things. For you have died, and your life is now hidden with Christ in God. When Christ, who is your life, appears, then you also will appear with Him in glory. Put to death, therefore, whatever belongs to your earthly nature (Col. 3:1-5).

Obviously Paul was not writing about physical death, but about death to the powers of sin and to our old way of living. The message is clear. We are not waiting to die, we have already died.

God has always called believers to a life of faith and obedience and to setting their sights on a larger picture than this world has to offer. This is hope at work. Through the sacrifice of Christ, we have died to the things of this world, and we are called to set our minds on things above.

My having cancer is not just some strange happening. I am merely experiencing a consequence of life which is, in some form or fashion, a part of everyone's experience. I am not suddenly in danger of dying, I have already died. My life is not measured in days or years in this world, it is already immeasureably eternal.

I know this may seem like I'm spiritualizing pain or making light of the suffering that goes along with dying. What I intend to do is show that hope—the real hope—gives an eternal perspective to even our deepest sorrows. We are going home, and what we have learned and how we have served God here does make a difference.

When Paul wrote his second epistle to the Corinthians, he encouraged them with this very thought. He said that our bodies are merely tents, not our permanent homes, and that we groan, longing to be clothed with our heavenly dwelling (2 Cor. 5:1-2).

Paul goes on to explain:

> We are always confident and know that as long as we are at home in the body we are away from the Lord. We live by faith, not by sight. We are confident, I say, and would prefer to be away from the body and at home with the Lord. So we make it our goal to please Him, whether we are at home in the body or away from it (2 Cor. 5:6-9).

Perhaps you can see, now, why it seems so strange to me for believers to make such a fuss over physical healing. It is not that I think such healing is insignificant (I will discuss this whole matter in a later chapter), I just don't think it is the most wonderful nor the most necessary display of God's power and grace.

We live in a body here on this earth for a time, but the end of that body is merely the beginning of "the life that is truly life" (1 Tim. 6:17-19).

When my uncle died, I learned even more clearly that this world is not my home. I am a pilgrim passing through on my way to the place I know as "home, sweet home."

So, what do we tell people about hope? Can a person who is dying really lose hope? Do our faces have to say, "How tragic this is," rather than "Welcome home"?

The whole essence of hope lies in grasping that which can never perish, spoil, or fade. We are eternally alive in Christ.

Questions to Consider

1. Have you ever lost someone you love to death? If so, how has it changed your understanding of heaven? Of hope?
2. How can the reality of heaven help you, right now, in whatever struggles you are facing? How does the example of the believers described in Hebrews 11 help you?
3. Identify and talk about those people in your life whom you see living with an eternal perspective.
4. What are the obstacles that make it difficult for a Christian to really live by faith and hope?
5. What do you think was going on in Paul's life when he penned the second letter to the Corinthians? Why do you suppose he understood so much about eternity?

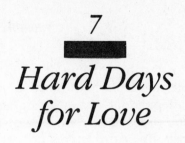

7

Hard Days for Love

"The hardest thing for me is so many caring, well-wishing friends saying how good I look and how well I am walking, when I want to scream, 'I'm not walking well, and I don't know if I ever will! I'm so slow. I hate having to think about every step I take!' It seems as if nobody wants to listen to how I feel about what happened to me. They just want to pat me on the back and breathe a sigh of relief that they don't have to worry anymore. Then I have guilty feelings for feeling this way about people who are being so nice to me and for being depressed when I am lucky."[1]
                                                    —Marilee Dunker

Seasons of Love

One of the most wonderful yet most difficult things about suffering is the relationships that ebb and flow throughout its course. The words above of Marilee Dunker accurately reflect the struggle that most people in pain experience with family and friends.

It is glorious to care for a person in his or her need, and

it is terribly difficult at the same time. We are proud people, particularly those of us who have been taught to be independent. We make a great effort to care for ourselves and to make sure we are not a burden on anyone else. We also prefer that others not place too much of their burden on us. When we are young and healthy, we can't imagine being incapacitated and needing someone's help just to go to the bathroom or to eat. We can't imagine anything taking from us our physical or emotional well-being and independence, but those circumstances do come—and they test us all as we pass through the seasons of love.

Shared Burdens

The most obvious concept about relationships and suffering is that shared burdens are lighter burdens. How many times have you watched someone struggle to lift a load alone, when a simple, "please help me" would make all the difference?

It's easy to romanticize the past and think it better than it actually was, but I do wonder if friendships were closer and suffering handled more candidly in days gone by. Did believers in the early church suffer with one another, even when it caused the body of Christ hardship?

Love is the trademark of the believer, but it isn't always easy to know how to muster up the courage to love for one more day.

Paul wrote the Galatians a seemingly contradictory message about burden-bearing. In the space of just a few verses, he instructed the members of the church about two different aspects of the issue.

"Carry each other's burdens," Paul writes, "and in this way you will fulfill the law of Christ" (Gal. 6:2). Then just a few verses later he adds, "each one should carry his own load" (Gal. 6:5).

It took me awhile to understand what Paul was trying to say. We think in terms of black and white, right and wrong, one way or the other; but Scripture often teaches from a different viewpoint.

These verses tell us that we must carry our own burden, and we must bear each other's loads. Shared burdens are lighter burdens—for both the sufferer and the friend.

We find the same principle at work in Solomon's words of wisdom:

> Two are better than one, because they have a good return for their work: If one falls down, his friend can help him up. But pity the man who falls and has no one to help him up! Also, if two lie down together, they will keep warm. But how can one keep warm alone? Though one may be overpowered, two can defend themselves. A cord of three strands is not quickly broken" (Ecc. 4:9-12).

Obviously, the sharing of burdens makes some kind of sense—that is, as long as the one with the burden doesn't completely unload. Two are stronger than one, but both must participate. When both are involved, they provide for one another the encouragement to carry on.

I have a mental picture of how this shared suffering works. Imagine a group of friends climbing a mountain together. Each carries a load of supplies, but no one is overburdened. As they climb, they come to a particularly difficult spot. Instead of shedding their burdens under the strain, each person slips a hand under his neighbor's pack and lifts—just a bit—to help make the load more bearable.

No one person can carry everyone's pack, for the weight would be intolerable. Neither should all the climbers maintain their independence, offering characteristic untruths like, "I don't need any help," or, "I'm fine!"

No matter what happens to us, we must pay attention to this twofold message found in Galatians. We must bear the crosses that God gives us to bear, for He asks nothing of us that we are unable to handle. He merely asks that we trust

Him to provide the very strength that's required to do the job.

On the other hand, we are to love one another and to be concerned with each other's needs. Scripture is filled with teaching after teaching about the working together of God's people. For someone to try lifting a heavy load alone is unnecessary when the body of Christ is around.

Jethro's Wisdom

When Moses began his term as Israel's leader, he was so scared that he tried to talk God out of giving him the job. He tried everything from "They won't believe me" (Ex. 4:1) to, "I've never been good with words" (Ex. 4:10). Much to Moses' dismay, however, the Lord was not convinced of his incompetence.

By the time Israel had passed through the Red Sea unscathed, there was no stopping Moses. He almost single-handedly led the Israelites through the wilderness, becoming a person of deep commitment to responsibility.

Then one day Jethro visited Moses. He was a wise man, and as he watched his son-in-law at work, he knew it was time to give some fatherly advice. Scripture records Jethro's conversation with Moses in the Book of Exodus.

> "What is this you are doing for the people? Why do you alone sit as judge, while all these people stand around you from morning till evening?"

> Moses answered him, "Because the people come to me to seek God's will. Whenever they have a dispute, it is brought to me, and I decide between the parties and inform them of God's decrees and laws."

> Moses' father-in-law replied, "What you are doing is not good. You and these people who come

to you will only wear yourselves out. The work is too heavy for you; you cannot handle it alone. Listen now to me and I will give you some advice, and may God be with you. You must be the people's representative before God and bring their disputes to Him. Teach them the decrees and laws, and show them the way to live and the duties they are to perform. But select capable men from all the people—men who fear God, trustworthy men who hate dishonest gain—and appoint them as officials over thousands, hundreds, fifties, and tens. Have them serve as judges for the people at all times, but have them bring every difficult case to you: The simple cases they can decide themselves. That will make your load lighter, because they will share it with you. If you do this and God so commands, you will be able to stand the strain, and all these people will go home satisfied."

Moses listened to his father-in-law and did everything he said (Ex. 18:14-24).

The principle is sound. When we try to carry all of the load by ourselves, we miss the privilege of seeing the body of Christ work together. And if we try to avoid carrying our own loads, we miss the growth that God has in store for us. God has designed a balanced, effective body.

Hard Days for Love

When we thought I had only a few months to live, the loving was easy. People went out of their way to help me up stairs or shop for my necessities or spend time listening to my songs and praises. It was a special time for me, and I will never forget the love which so many generously gave me.

When the nine months was over, however, and the bookend of death was, again, off in the distance, friendships were not quite as simple as they had been at first. People began to want a break from living the daily grind of my illness, and I could not blame them. It is hard to be friends with someone who is dying or experiencing chronic pain.

A chronic sufferer must handle physical and mental weariness, address emotional changes and needs, evaluate spiritual questions and growth—and all of these things take up a tremendous amount of time and energy. In short, we who are afflicted with various pains live life in a very intense way. This can be exhausting for those close to us.

One day, my ministry partner and I were doing one of our programs for a large, local church. We were sitting on stools, as usual, sharing about the difficulties of the cancer, when my partner gave a spontaneous evaluation: "Shelley is dying, but it's killing me!"

Fortunately, most of the people in the audience knew us, so they were not offended by the seeming irreverence of the remark. I was certainly not offended. He was right. It is not easy to die right along with someone else.

We generally protect ourselves, if possible, from real suffering. I have friends who refuse to watch certain documentaries or follow world disasters because it is too depressing to see another's struggle. Suffering certainly can be depressing, but it's also a reality of life.

Those who stay for a time with Mother Teresa usually speak of the horrendous emotional adjustment they must make those first few hours of watching people die. Holding a starving child or seeing an adult, emaciated and ravaged by a fever, can break anyone's heart.

We weep to hear of another's pain, but to actually live through that pain with our loved one, day in and day out, is an exhausting strain. It is said, and rightly so, that an individual who is ill often outlives the capacity of friends and family to bear the burden.

It is easier for me to write about this struggle today, after I have lived through it myself and counseled many others in their struggles. It was not easy to understand during the first year of my own illness.

Many times I wanted to cry to my friends, "Don't you care? Can't you see that I need you here to help me right now? How can you go out to a movie or watch television or leave for a party? I'm sick!" The person who is ill cannot get away to a movie or a nice restaurant. I used to wish I had a zipper on my body so that I could leave the burden behind—just for a few moments.

Suffering is trying, not only for the patient, but also for those who are watching and waiting and trying to meet the conglomeration of needs. It took time for me to realize that although my friends had run out of energy, they had not run out of love. And it took time for them to learn to speak with me openly about their fears and needs. We had to understand each other.

Though I will talk later in the book about many of the issues facing families and friends, I want to discuss here the need for treating the problem of chronic suffering realistically, with confidence and, above all else, with honesty.

Facing and dealing with the reality of physical or emotional illness can become a divisive puzzle for patients and caregivers if those involved fail to approach it candidly. We fear naked disclosure, but this is the best way not only to deal with the illness, but also to make it through the problem in one piece.

From the Standpoint of Family and Friends

One of the biggest steps which family and friends must take is the step of accepting the reality of the struggle. Such acceptance does not come easily. It is difficult to see someone we love trapped inside a body that will no longer function or plagued by emotional turmoil. We want to pretend the illness isn't that bad, or convince ourselves that the problem will soon go away. When we ignore the reality of the predicament, however, we do ourselves and the sufferer a real disservice.

As Jesus approached His final days, He tried to warn the disciples of His upcoming suffering and death, but they would not hear of such a thing!

> From that time on Jesus began to explain to His disciples that He must go to Jerusalem and suffer many things at the hands of the elders, chief priests and teachers of the law, and that He must be killed and on the third day be raised to life.

> Peter took Him aside and began to rebuke Him. "Never, Lord!" he said. "This shall never happen to you!" (Matt. 16:21-22)

Can you imagine such a conversation? When I picture it, all I can do is smile. Peter not only didn't hear the best part (the Resurrection!), but he also thought he could determine history and control the destiny of our Lord. I would love to have seen the look of surprise on Peter's face when Jesus responded with these words:

> "Get behind me, Satan! You are a stumbling block to Me; you do not have in mind the things of God, but the things of man" (Matt. 16:23).

I don't think Peter understood why Jesus was so upset. From the disciple's perspective, he was offering to protect His Lord. What was Peter missing?

As family and friends of a person who is ill, we are sometimes like Peter—we do not want to see what is really happening to our loved one. We want to believe that God will restore health or that the medicine will make things better. We want to believe that life will soon return to "normal."

Wanting a loved one to get better is not wrong, but it is

dangerous to refuse to accept and deal with the reality of a person's situation. We need to open those lines of communication and face the pain together. If we do not, we leave ourselves open to unresolved feelings of guilt and regret.

When we read how Jesus prepared the disciples but how little they seemed to understand about His arrest, trial, and crucifixion, we can see that the Twelve were not really tuned in to that part of Jesus' ministry. They chose, instead, to deny the very purpose for His coming.

It is hard to face the prospect of a loved one's death. It is hard to imagine that one we love may actually live in pain for the rest of his or her time in this world. It is hard to watch someone we love lose weight or the ability to remember or sensitivity or zeal or that rosy blush of the cheeks or that gleam in the eye. We want to believe the pain will go away, so we pretend that all is well.

For the first three or four years of my pain, people would try to advise or console me by saying that I just needed to rest or learn meditation. They would say that vitamins would do the trick or that exercise would take the pain away. They meant well, but I couldn't understand why everyone wanted to avoid the pain except me.

I can't count the number of people I have counseled who have said to me, "My mother is ill, but she can't talk about the illness," or, "We'd tell my husband the truth, but we don't want him to lose hope."

Most of the time, it is the family and friends who are afraid of the discussions—the loved ones who are afraid of losing hope. The dying or suffering person can usually handle the reality of the situation. How much easier it is if the caregivers can also handle the dilemma intimately and realistically.

As bystanders, we make it harder on ourselves and the patient when we try to pretend or keep "a stiff upper lip." Generally, if we can cry and talk with the sufferer and deal openly with the realities of the problem, strength will come as it's needed, one day at a time.

From the Perspective of the Sufferer

For the sufferer, honesty plays a bit of a different role. It can be extremely frustrating to sense that our loved ones are afraid of talking about our problems. Ignoring the obvious hurts.

I have had friends come into my hospital room with flowers and smiles and light discussion. "You look wonderful today," they say, as they open the blinds or rearrange the flowers. I know they are trying to bring cheer to the room, but I also know that I don't look wonderful. It is awkward to make superficial conversation when much deeper issues are really at stake. When I sense that the visitor is uncomfortable with my pain, I usually feel responsible to try and lessen that person's load. Before you know it, I am doing the cheering.

We who are ill do not need someone to fix our problem. The ultimate fixing lies in the hands of our resurrected Lord, and we are delighted to leave it there. We really just want to be close to the ones we love, and to share the journey with them.

As Jesus approached the moment of His arrest, He took Peter, James, and John with Him to pray for the courage to face that event:

> He took Peter and the two sons of Zebedee along with Him, and He began to be sorrowful and troubled. Then He said to them, "My soul is overwhelmed with sorrow to the point of death. Stay here and keep watch with Me" (Matt. 26:37-38).

The three friends could do nothing to change Jesus' struggles or take away the burden He faced, but they could share that burden by keeping watch with Him, by joining in His sorrow and prayers. That was all He asked.

Going a little farther, He fell with His face to the ground and prayed, "My Father, if it is possible, may this cup be taken from Me. Yet not as I will, but as You will." Then He returned to His disciples and found them sleeping. "Could you men not keep watch with Me for one hour?" He asked Peter. "Watch and pray so that you will not fall into temptation. The Spirit is willing, but the body is weak" (Matt. 26:39-41).

I can understand a bit of Jesus' struggle. I have felt, at times, as if my friends were somehow incapable of feeling with me or sharing my anguish. They seem to fall asleep at some of my most lonely moments.

Jesus didn't want the disciples to fix His problem, He just wanted them to share His burden. He did not ask them to pray that God would change the plan, He just wanted them to stay awake.

The person who is suffering wants friends and family to listen, to care, to talk about the pain, to sit by the bed for awhile, even if there's little to say.

It is an uncomfortable position, to be beside someone you love and not be able to ease the pain. And yet to avoid the reality of that pain only makes it harder to bear for everyone. I believe that strength flows through the stream of honest loving confrontation. If you are weary from caring for your loved one and need a break, say so. If you are afraid of watching someone you love die, tell that person.

If you are the patient and you just want your friends and family members to talk to you, ask them. If you want them to sit and hold your hand, say so. If you are afraid, talk about the fear. We often let a tough situation get the best of us because we avoid being honest.

I am not telling you that honesty will always be easy. It won't. Honesty may bring some tears today or a few weeks of insecurity, but in the long run, it is a much healthier way to deal with the sadness and grief which accompany physical pain, emotional illness, or death. We can face anything with God's grace and the love and support of one another.

In a world in which control is the name of the game, we must remember that life cannot always be controlled. We have the responsibility to accept what God allows and to help others do the same. As Paul reminds us, we must carry our own load, and we must also carry each other's burdens.

We find it difficult to yield control to that which seems to be an enemy, but we must remember that death is no longer the enemy and that pain is used by God to mold and mature us, developing within us a faith that is purer than gold (1 Peter 1:3-7).

These are hard days for love. We feel helpless when there is little we can do. Just remember, as you walk through the pain with those you love, God will provide the strength.

Questions to Consider

1. What has been the most difficult pain you have personally had to bear (physical, emotional, or spiritual)?
2. What did you need the most from family and friends during your pain?
3. Try to imagine someone you love being sick or in need. What would be your first reaction in trying to help that person? What might you do to better help that person now?
4. If you are ill or in pain right now, what are some things you wish your family and friends understood about you?
5. How has God given you strength in your moments of greatest need?

8

Pain As Companion

My servant, I have come into the house—
I, who know pain's extremity so well
That there can never be the need to tell
His power to make the flesh and spirit quail.
Have I not felt the scourge, the thorn, the nail?
And I, his Conqueror, am in the house.
Let not your heart be troubled, do not fear.
Why shouldst thou, child of Mine, if I am here?
My touch will heal thy songbird's broken wing
And he shall have a braver song to sing." [1]

—Amy Carmichael

Acquainted with Grief

I know you have heard the story of Job—the man who suffered unspeakable pain with God's consent. You have probably heard his story more times than you can count. Still, I don't know how to discuss suffering without visiting a man who was well acquainted with grief. Job has much to teach us on the topic.

In the opening verses of the Book of Job, we read about Satan presenting himself to God after "roaming through the earth and going back and forth in it" (Job 1:7). We don't know just what Satan had in mind, but we do know how God answered the fallen angel: "Have you considered My servant Job? There is no one on earth like him; he is blameless and upright, a man who fears God and shuns evil" (Job 1:8).

It would seem that Satan had a bit of wanderlust that day. Perhaps he was seeking someone to devour, and God made the choice for him. It is hard for us to imagine God volunteering Job for such a position, but that is exactly what He did. God knew that Job's love for Him wasn't based on the possessions and positions He had given Job. Satan wasn't convinced.

A heated round of spiritual warfare began. While Job was at his house one day, Satan struck his children, his herds, his flocks, and his servants until all that Job held dear had been destroyed. When Job heard the news, we are told that he tore his robe, shaved his head, and worshiped God (Job 1:20). "Naked I came from my mother's womb," Job wept, "and naked I will depart. The Lord gave and the Lord has taken away; may the name of the Lord be praised" (Job 1:21).

It's appropriate for us to pause for a moment to consider the words we've just read. It is almost beyond my imagination to think that a man who had just lost everything would choose, as his first act, to worship God. I am accustomed to hearing people complain in angry and bitter tones over far less loss. Rarely do I see people worship God in the wake of their pain. But Job was a man who loved God, and he managed to hold onto that love in the midst of his loss.

When Satan saw that his plan had not achieved the desired results, he returned to the presence of God for part two of the spiritual skirmish. God again praised Job, and this time Satan targeted Job's physical body. "Skin for skin!" Satan exclaimed. "A man will give all he has for his own life. But stretch out your hand and strike his flesh and bones, and he will surely curse you to your face" (Job 2:4-5).

While Job was still grieving over the loss of his children and livelihood, Satan afflicted his body with sores that extended from the top of his head to the bottom of his feet. The agony must have seemed unbearable, but we find that in all this, Job did not sin (Job 2:7-10).

God really is in charge of the world, our lives, and our pain. We make ignorant choices, we sin and fall short of His ideal, we avoid growth, we choose the more comfortable route; but we are still actors in an eternal play—one which we cannot yet see.

Though suffering can be the result of God's discipline, it can also be the result of events and relationships and purposes which are not made clear to man. Often we are too quick to assign cause to the effect. As believers, we are not removed from pain and suffering. Instead, we take comfort in the fact that God accompanies us through the pain and suffering. We are God's children, and He has a plan and a purpose for each and every one of us.

Job was not in pain because of his sin, although his friends would try to convict him of such a connection. Job was not in pain because Satan tricked God and got away with the trick. Job was not in pain because he was a bad guy and God wanted to teach him a lesson. Job was not in pain as the result of some freakish event of nature that was out of God's control.

Though all these excuses sound silly, they are, nonetheless, representative of excuses I hear all the time. We tell ourselves that pain only comes to those who somehow deserve to suffer or those whose faith is not strong enough to provide relief. This was simply not the case with Job, nor is it the case with countless others who have known suffering.

Job's story has been my strength in the years I've lived with pain. It not only encourages me in my suffering, but it also reveals how God works in our lives in mysterious yet sovereign ways. Pain is never without purpose, and we are never without God, even in the midst of pain. He knows what He is doing.

I will leave the detailed unfolding of Job's life for another book, but the end of the story is something I want to explore. It reveals pain as comrade rather than intruder.

God thought Job worthy of the trial. He believed that Job could finish the race and hear, "Well done, My good and faithful servant." I think that is exactly what Job heard the day he faced God.

As recorded in the Bible, Job worked through his grief, step by step. He said, "I wish I had never been born," and he begged God to have mercy and leave him to die with his wounds. Job also listened to the insensitive advice of friends who had once seemed to know him.

"Where was God all this time?" we might ask. "Couldn't God have given Job a hint of the conversation that had taken place in heaven? Couldn't God have told Job that the advice of his friends was invalid?"

Yes, God could have done those things, but He chose to wait patiently for just the right moment to show Job a purpose for his pain. Job asked God question after question throughout his days of anguish and, finally we read that God answered Job out of a storm.

I like to imagine that Job was listening to "round three" of his friends at the time, when all at once he began to hear the Lord's words roll out with the thunder: "Who is this that darkens My counsel with words without knowledge? Brace yourself like a man; I will question you, and you shall answer Me" (Job 38:2-3).

God continued to pose questions to Job—questions no man could possibly answer.

• "Where were you when I laid the earth's foundation?" (Job 38:4)

• "Have you ever given orders to the morning or shown the dawn its place?" (Job 38:12)

• "Do you give the horse his strength or clothe his neck

with a flowing mane?" (Job 39:19)

I think that God did for Job the same thing He is doing for me. Through the suffering, God taught Job about Himself. He taught Job that He is trustworthy and completely in control. He taught Job that He is the Creator and the Life-giver and the all-powerful Sustainer of everything He has created.

Instead of saying, "Job, I know your life has really been tough since I let Satan take away all your treasures," God turned Job's eyes to Himself—to the eternal. He never even mentioned Job's loss.

Somehow, everything else comes into perspective when God is the measuring line. Everything else makes sense when we view it through the eyes of the Creator Himself.

After hearing God speak, Job gave a reply that I continue to make my own.

> "I know that You can do all things; no plan of Yours can be thwarted. . . . Surely I spoke of things I did not understand, things too wonderful for me to know. . . . My ears had heard of You but now my eyes have seen You" (Job 42:1-5).

Job was still in physical pain when he responded to God. He was still without family, friends, possessions, and the respect of the townspeople. But he had the most wonderful gift of all—a greater awareness of his Father.

If we could ask Job, today, whether the end result was worth the pain, I believe he would say, "Absolutely! I learned to see my God."

The Presence of Pain

Living with physical pain is a difficult responsibility. I can honestly say that I no longer remember what it was like to really feel good. I know that I did feel good at one time. In fact, I spent most of my life in excellent physical health. I had nothing to complain about until I was 28, and for that

I am more thankful now than I ever was before. Now I wake up every morning with the acute awareness of pain, and every night I close my eyes with a heavy sigh. Pain is my comrade throughout every hour of every day.

One of the most jolting realizations about physical pain is that it doesn't kill you! Instead, a person in chronic pain may live with that pain for a number of years. That is a frightening thought.

Unfortunately, many Christians in the United States say that no one needs to live in pain. How cruel those words can sound when they are spoken without firsthand knowledge. I never understood pain until it became part of my life, and it remains the thing I find most difficult to convey to others. Either people have not experienced pain, or they don't want to understand its reality. That makes the explaining hard.

I believe that pain is a gift—a challenging one. It can raise us to the heights of joy, or it can pull us down to the depths of despair.

If we view pain as an enemy rather than a comrade, we will come to walk with desperation. If we hate suffering's presence, we will come to hate our life as well. Many people in pain hide themselves behind walls and wait— wait for the moment the pain will be over. Few days are longer than a day lived despising one's own existence.

If we view pain as a companion, we can begin to look through suffering's eyes at a world which lives in pain. We begin to see what God sees and learn to care the way He cares. I have met few people who have chosen this route, but their joy is undeniable. Their eyes gleam with a grateful awareness of God's love and a sense of perspective.

I believe pain is a gift because of what it teaches the believer, and it is that gift I would like to unfold in the remaining pages of this chapter.

Most of my lessons have been gleaned from enduring physical pain, but that is not the only suffering from which we can learn—nor is it necessarily the worst kind of suffering. Pain comes in all shapes and sizes, and each is allowed in our lives for a purpose.

The Character of Pain

When I am teaching on the value of pain, I usually begin by asking the audience two questions: "Would you like your children to have faith, character, perseverance, discipline, and maturity? Would you like your children to really understand hope?"

Almost every parent I've met replies, "Certainly! Those are important qualities for my child to develop." And I agree.

According to Scripture, these are indeed some of the most important qualities we can develop, but they are also a by-product of suffering. Yes, it is true. Suffering, in its many forms, produces the eternal and internal qualities that each of us hungers to have and to bequeath to our children. (See Job 42:5; Rom. 5:1-5; Phil. 1:29; 3:10; Heb. 11; James 1:2-4; 1 Peter 1:3-9.)

As you might imagine, I have had countless conversations with those who say that God does not want me to suffer. I will cover this attitude more in depth in the chapter on healing, but it needs to be addressed briefly here as well.

Suffering is seen as a negative experience by most people, so we do our best to explain it away or pretend it doesn't have to exist. We don't like the implications of living with something for which there is no end or solution in sight.

We know certain types of suffering are unavoidable, but we still do our best to keep them far away. Let me illustrate.

Few of us would argue that suffering as a martyr for the sake of the Gospel is anything short of godly suffering. After all, men and women in both the Old and New Testament days were asked to participate in such sacrifice. And

we all know the stories of missionaries who have courageously given their lives to spread the Gospel. Yet, while
we commend such people for their faith, we also pray that
martyrdom will not be demanded of us or our children.
We admire that kind of suffering, but we keep it at a
distance.

We must remember that suffering is part of the process
of learning. We are not alone in our pain—God is present.
He knows our every need, so we need not fear the unfolding of the plan.

A Personal Look

My physical pain began just a few months after my first
surgery for cancer. At first we thought the cancer had returned, but the tests showed no presence of the disease.
The pain was a result of the surgical procedures—a pain
that would probably remain.

As the days and weeks went by and the pain continued,
I cried to God late into the night, "Please not this. First
You ask me to die; then You leave me here when I'm
finally excited about coming home; and now You want me
to live here indefinitely with physical pain! How long can
this go on?" Finally, exhaustion would lull me to sleep. I
was searching for some response from God, but I could
not hear His reply—at least not yet.

The struggle went on for months. I was living with pain
and expecting God to take it away any moment. I imagine
He must have tired of my pleas, for every night was a
repeat of the last: "Please, God, I just have to sleep. Do
something to make it stop. I can't live this way."

The days were easier than the nights. At least during the
day I was traveling or speaking somewhere and the time
passed more quickly. At night, the minutes seemed like
hours as I listened to the clock keep its never-ending vigil.

I was given medication to help take the edge off the
pain, but it too had its drawbacks. It made me feel nause-

ated and sleepy all the time, yet if I cut down on the dosage, the pain became too hard to bear. It took months to strike the right balance between medication and side effects.

Part of my pain during that period of my life was mental anguish. The *whys* bothered me; but, more than that, I couldn't seem to make the doctors understand the condition of my body. It is hard to verbally describe pain, and I felt as if my doctors really didn't believe my suffering was *that* bad.

I thought I was at the end of my rope when God finally gave me a lift one night. I had been on pain medication for a year at that point and had grown accustomed to little sleep. That particular evening I prayed, "OK, Father, if You aren't going to help me sleep, then at least entertain me! I'm probably the only person in this hemisphere talking to You at this hour, so I expect you have a little extra time."

I knew I was being a bit careless with God in that prayer, but He answered me—right there on the spot. I didn't see any visions or dream any dreams, I just sensed God's gentle urging to recount the changes in my life during that year of living with pain.

I realized I had become more loving and compassionate than I had ever been before. I used to think people should be able to handle their pain, but that year, arthritis or migraine headaches or acute back pain brought a new reaction of empathy from me.

I realized I had become more patient. I really didn't have any choice! There were days when my body would not cooperate and other days when my strength seemed to disappear. I had been forced to learn to nap when I was tired and to say no to activities that might drain me. I had learned to treat people in pain with patience because I needed patience to cope with my own suffering.

I noticed that my faith had grown stronger in those nights and days of depending on God for rest and strength. Though I had always needed God, I had never known how much I needed Him until pain took its place in my life. I needed Him to make it through the day and the night. Such dependence did wonders for my faith.

I realized that my ability to comfort others had taken on new proportions. I had learned to do for hurting people what God was doing for me. I could cry with, or sit with, or pray for, or listen to, or just hold a person who was suffering.

God responded to my challenge that night by showing me all that He'd been doing in my heart during that year of pain. It dawned on me that God had been molding me into the very person I had prayed to become—He had just used a different tool than I'd expected.

Sometimes our pain is brought on by our own sins. Sometimes our pain is a result of the sins of another person. Sometimes suffering is the result of living under someone else's command. And sometimes suffering comes simply because we live in a fallen world.

We rarely know the reason for suffering, but if we trust God and believe what He has told us in His Word, we can be sure that He will use the pain for both His benefit and ours.

My pain has been the companion that has taken me to God. Without the suffering, I would have been too young and too proud and too certain of my own abilities to really open up my eyes and see my Heavenly Father. Oh, I had heard of Him, as had Job. I had professed His name from the time I was nine and then taught more Bible studies than I can now count. But the way I began to see Him in the midst of my pain was something new.

Now, I need Him and His grace, and I adore being weak when He is strong. I continue to learn to trust Him and His will even when it hurts me for the moment. And I think about Him and about His perspective as I run the races of this life.

It has taken suffering for me to understand what is truly significant in this world. We want to possess and conquer, trying to gain our significance from that which we can control. We imagine God's ways to be our own, but in doing so, we miss Him.

I am learning, in these years with pain, a little bit more about the grace, forgiveness, love, patience, endurance, and comfort which so characterize God's nature. I am learning a little more about who He is and what He desires. I am learning that we are here to please God, honor Him, and abide by His plan. We are here to love Him and His people and to give up our lives for that which is truly life. This is significance.

If you had offered me complete healing and restoration in 1982, I would have taken it gladly. In fact, many people petitioned God for just such a miracle. Now, looking back, I would choose to live life exactly as God has allowed. Paul expressed my own thoughts so well in his second letter to the Corinthians.

> Three times I pleaded with the Lord to take [my thorn] away from me. But He said to me, "My grace is sufficient for you, for My power is made perfect in weakness." Therefore, I will boast all the more gladly about my weaknesses, so that Christ's power may rest on me. That is why, for Christ's sake, I delight in weaknesses, in insults, in hardships, in persecutions, in difficulties. For when I am weak, then I am strong" (2 Cor. 12:8-10).

If we will open our eyes to see God in the suffering, then the journey of pain holds meaning and purpose and great joy.

Purpose in the Pain

Although I have focused on physical pain in this chapter, I know that most of us also undergo emotional and mental pain. Often when we hurt physically, we must also deal with the emotional stress and vice versa. When our mind is burdened, our body often sends messages of similar despair. When the emotions find no rest, neither can the mind.

Regardless of the type of pain, the lesson is the same: God has designed purpose in our pain, and we need not fear its discovery. The treasures of pain are eternal, and they serve us well in the journey.

If I could offer one piece of advice for those who suffer pain, it would be this: do not despise your own pain. When we hate our own reality, we quickly find ourselves void of the capacity to deal with the suffering.

I know that what I am asking is difficult. Most people who suffer try to avoid its acceptance for a long, long time. They search for cures, relief, reasons, and solutions, but they soon become weary.

I am not asking you to avoid possible solutions. I am merely urging you to begin with acceptance, and to bathe your path with understanding. We cannot grow when we refuse to accept our situation. We cannot mature when we despise the process God has chosen.

Questions to Consider

1. Are you afraid of suffering? If so, why? What kind of suffering causes you the most fear?
2. Look back on those times when you were in great pain, physically or emotionally. What did you learn through those times?
3. What are some of the questions you would like to ask God someday?
4. If pain is your companion, where do you need to walk with pain right now?
5. Think of five people you know who are currently experiencing some sort of pain. How can you help them to better understand their pain?

9

Clay in the Potter's Hand

"Many of us try to get out of pain as fast as we can, so that we can be more 'useful' to God. Yet God reminds us again and again throughout Scripture that His greatest treasure fills earthen vessels, in order to show that the transcendent power belongs to God and not to us. In our weakness, we are strong. Earthen vessels are God's first choice. Let God fill you just as you are. Let Him touch you and use you in your fragile and fallible state."[1]

–Tim Hansel

The Potter's House

One of my favorite passages of Scripture is the story of Jeremiah the prophet. Jeremiah had been faithful to God for years and had experienced much anguish in his endeavor to reach the Israelites with God's message. As was their custom, the Israelites refused to listen—a condition which left the prophet very discouraged.

One day, God sent Jeremiah on a journey: "Go down to the potter's house, and there I will give you My message"

(Jer. 18:2). I can picture Jeremiah cautiously approaching a house and then peering through the window.

> So I went down to the potter's house, and I saw him working at the wheel. But the pot he was shaping from the clay was marred in his hands; so the potter formed it into another pot, shaping it as seemed best to him. Then the word of the Lord came to me: "O House of Israel, can I not do with you as this potter does?" declares the Lord. "Like clay in the hand of the potter, so are you in My hand, O house of Israel" (Jer. 18:3-7).

I am sure that the first vessel made by the potter looked fine to Jeremiah. The untrained eye is not able to see that which the craftsman can discern. Yet the potter destroyed the vessel with his own hands! He took that fine composition and began to remake and reform the piece of clay until it was exactly the way he intended it to be.

When I was in grade school, I made a ceramic bowl in art class one day. I took great care in forming my bowl, but I grew impatient with the process. The teacher told us that all of the bubbles had to be worked out of the clay, but that took time. I wanted to get to the fun part. I wanted to paint my bowl blue and green and watch it bake in the kiln.

When the time came for the kiln to be opened and our pieces retrieved, mine was not there. I couldn't understand what had happened. I had placed the bowl in the oven myself! The teacher felt sorry for me, I could tell. I could also tell that she knew exactly what had happened.

"You did not work the bubbles out," she told me. "If there are bubbles in the clay, then the bowl is imperfect and it cannot withstand the heat of the kiln. Let's try again."

Those words spoken by my childhood art teacher illustrate the concept of God as the Master Potter. If we are patient and wise, we will not only sit still for the molding, but we will relish the care He takes with each creation. He is making of us exactly what He desires.

He has taken me through some molding that has been quite painful, and there will probably be still more of that painful process in store. I can see, however, that the end result of this pain is good. God is making me into His image. And that's what I've always wanted.

He is teaching me to love, and to cry, and to hunger for righteousness. He is teaching me to count it all loss for the sake of knowing Christ Jesus my Lord. He is teaching me to depend upon Him and to trust His ways. He is teaching me to plant seeds of His love in the lives of others.

In 1982, I could not understand how any good could possibly come out of cancer, particularly in the life of a 28-year-old. I spent hours trying to figure out what God could possibly accomplish through such a mess.

Now, I have a hard time seeing anything but the good. He has accomplished more in me and through me than I ever thought possible—and all because He cared enough to work out the bubbles so that I could withstand the kiln of suffering.

My prayer for my fellow Christians is the same one I pray for myself. Oh, that we, like Paul, would "want to know Christ and the power of His resurrection and the fellowship of sharing in His sufferings, becoming like Him in His death, and so, somehow, to attain to the resurrection from the dead" (Phil. 3:10-11).

It isn't easy to lose to find, to give up to gain, or to die to live. It isn't easy to release the reins of our lives to God. The result, however, is all that we ever dreamed faith could be. We are clay that is being carefully shaped by the Potter—a skillful artisan.

Working Out the Bubbles

Everyone was surprised when my cancer did not return. For several years we kept expecting it to appear in X rays, but it did not. By 1986, the doctors felt good about my prognosis and so did my family and friends. It seemed that God had something other than physical death in mind for me.

Physical pain remained my most difficult test. The medications worked for a time, but my body grew accustomed to the chemicals and it took more and more to achieve the desired result. I did not want to take large doses of narcotics forever, so I began to search for an alternate way to live with the pain.

In June of 1986 I made an appointment with a specialist and discovered a new method of pain control called an "epidural catheter." The catheter operates by anesthetizing the problem portion of the body, thus offering relief. I decided to take my chances.

I thought I was well prepared mentally for the procedure. The doctor would thread a small tube up the epidural space in my spinal column and then weave that tube under the skin to the front of my body, just above the waist. As I needed help for the pain, I would inject medication through the tube in front, and it would travel around my side, up the epidural space, and filter out into the problem areas. It sounded simple enough, and I was ready to try something new.

The procedure was successful from the medical standpoint. It took almost three hours, but the doctor was able to thread the tube with little difficulty. The hardest part was bringing the tube around my waist. The only way to accomplish such a feat is to make several incisions and then "sew" the tube around under the skin. Although I was sedated, the pain of the procedure itself was very real.

When I returned to the hospital room, I had to take the first lesson in giving myself injections. I don't know what I expected, but as the nurse unwrapped the bandage around my waist, I was horrified. The tube was larger than I thought it would be, and the way it sat on my stomach made me cry. I continued to have that reaction for several weeks because each time I looked in the mirror or tried to bathe, the contraption stared back in my face.

One of the difficult things about cancer and about surgery is the condition in which it leaves the body. I had several scars and a few "caves" in my chest area from the original surgery, and now this "thing" was so apparent. I felt sure everyone could see the apparatus under my clothing, and the thought was humbling. I went home from the hospital after several days, and began my new life with the catheter.

I had to be careful to keep the procedure as sterile as possible, and that worried me at first. The medicine had to be mixed in just the right way, and I had to make sure nothing touched the needle or the end of the tube during the injection.

The funniest ordeal was taking a bath without getting the catheter wet! One thing was certain: this new technique was far more entertaining than I'd imagined.

To make a long story short, that first catheter in 1986 soon gave way to seven more tubes and four unsuccessful attempts in the space of two years. Each surgery brought hope of more effective relief, yet the relief was always temporary. Sometimes the catheter lasted for only a few weeks; once it lasted for a whole five months! Whatever the time frame, it became apparent that the catheter was not a long-term solution to my problem. Finally, the doctors could no longer thread the tube up the epidural space, and the method became obsolete for me.

I wish I could count how many people have asked, "Why would you want something like that in your body?" For people who have not lived with pain, the nuisance of the catheter and the fact that it is so physically unattractive does not compute to usefulness.

People in pain, however, are way beyond the luxury of worrying about the outside. It is far more necessary to find some reprieve from the 24-hour visitor. Feeling relief from pain is worth the inconvenience, and definitely worth any physical unattractiveness that goes along with the relief.

I mention this process to you simply because I want you to know that I continue to struggle, daily, with the maturing process of God. I am not speaking to you from a one-time, quick, brush-with-pain perspective, but from a lasting journey with suffering.

I want you to see that the way we respond to the molding process of God makes all the difference. Life has continued to be painful for me, but God has continued to be faithful.

I think some people have been uncomfortable with my pain because they see their own frailty in me. Those with visible struggles remind us all of our weaknesses, and such a reminder is not often welcomed.

If I thought this were my glorified body, I'd be very discouraged. I believe, however, that it is only my "tent" and that the struggles with this tent teach me to separate the eternal from the temporal. That lesson is very important.

Into the Kiln Once Again

Normally, if a cancer patient can make it through five years without a recurrence, the doctors pronounce the cancer "no longer a serious threat."

As the "magic" year for cancer recovery approached, I seemed to be in good health.

The pain was still a battle, and I was on my third catheter at the time, but the overall picture looked promising from the medical standpoint. I was probably free from cancer, at least for the time being, and I could plan my days accordingly.

In January of 1987, I began to feel as if something was no longer fine in my body. The only way to detect my type of cancer is by CT scan, so I asked the doctor to schedule me for the test. I couldn't really explain my perception, it just seemed the pain had somehow changed.

I have tried to maintain a posture of joy throughout the illness, so it is difficult, at times, to get the attention of those who monitor my care. They agreed to run a scan, but I also knew they thought it unnecessary.

"Shelley, we got the results from the radiologist." The voice on the other end of the line seemed tense. "There are two spots visible on the scan, so we'll need to do a biopsy and see what they are."

Even though I had expected as much, I felt stunned. I knew the source of the spots, and many of the feelings I had experienced in October of 1982 returned in a rush.

I didn't want to go through that surgery again, but I knew that I had to do just that. A heavy sigh came over my whole body as I replaced the phone receiver. I well understood what was in store.

Four years and six months after the discovery of my cancer, I was headed for surgery again. The cancer had, indeed, recurred, and I was faced with a repeat performance of that which had turned my world upside down. I couldn't believe it was happening again.

In some ways the second time around would be easier. This time I would know what to ask for and what to expect, and I would understand the pain. In other ways, this second operation would be more difficult than the first because I *did* know what to expect. And I knew that I stood the chance of losing even more of that which was precious to me.

I had one prayer, as I faced the cancer a second time. "Father," I asked, "please help me to remember what I've been teaching others for the past four and a half years."

I had taught others about God's grace and love for nearly five years. I had told people how insignificant the earthly body is compared to the spiritual blessings of eternity. I had encouraged people that we need not fear that which God allows. And I had taught people about the all-sufficient grace of God and the hidden gifts of pain.

What if I weren't able to live those lessons? What if my

own situation proved harder than I could bear? What if my faith failed me and fear took control?

I felt as if this were my testing ground. I wanted to be able to apply, in the heat of the battle, the myriad of lessons I had learned and shared with others.

I knew before the surgery that there was a chance I would lose the right lung and pleural lining. There was no way to be certain ahead of time, but the doctor wanted to prepare me for that possibility.

A few days before my surgery I remember sitting in my music room, thinking about all the songs I had written and the pleasure that singing had brought me through the years. From the time I was a child, I had written music to soothe my heart in the various struggles of life. Perhaps singing would no longer be possible.

In an attempt to protect my treasured memories, I decided to record all the songs I had written. The event was wonderful! For two consecutive nights, I sang and played the guitar and called upon God's gracious gift that had been given to me for so many years.

Then, as if my life were on instant replay, I was wheeled into surgery early on the morning of March 30, 1987. The surgeon found three more tumors that day, and he removed part of another rib and a portion of my right lung. The entire lung and lining, however, had been spared.

The procedure was the same as my earlier surgery, and the reality of cancer was, once again, part of my life. This time, however, I knew from the moment I awoke that God had answered my prayer. The lessons He had taught me really do work; they are not theoretical. If we will trust God, even the most painful events have meaning and His blessing. I had taught about His grace and love, and I would be able to continue.

Our bodies are tents, but we are also the dwelling places of the Holy Spirit. Our bodies do fade, but with the fading of the temporal comes the glory of the eternal (2 Cor. 4:16; 5:1).

God uses us to bring glory to Himself, even when all that others see is a fading image of a once strong body. He is the Potter, and we are the clay.

A Building from God

A close friend of mine died of a brain tumor in the summer of 1989. He loved the Lord as much as anyone I've ever known, and we had the privilege of sharing with each other the comfort that only God can give. Tom was a man of faith, and that faith was reflected in the way that he died.

Only a short time before he went home, I sat beside Tom's bed with his wife. Tom was at the point of needing diapers and speaking in slow, deliberate syllables, but it did not stop him from wanting to talk about the Lord.

"Read me those verses about the tent," he requested. He could not remember the specifics of the passage, but he knew it applied to him:

> Now we know that if the earthly tent we live in is destroyed, we have a building from God, an eternal house in heaven, not built by human hands. Meanwhile we groan, longing to be clothed with our heavenly dwelling, because when we are clothed, we will not be found naked. For while we are in this tent, we groan and are burdened, because we do not wish to be unclothed but to be clothed with our heavenly dwelling, so that what is mortal may be swallowed up by life. Now it is God who has made us for this very purpose and has given us the Spirit as a deposit, guaranteeing what is to come (2 Cor. 5:1-5).

It is not easy for the healthy person to understand those words, but they are sweeter than honey to a person whose body is cracked and broken. Those of us who are ill *do* groan—and not just to be free from the pain, but to see Jesus.

"My tent is full of holes," Tom said, with the biggest smile I had seen on his face for awhile. "My tent is full of holes. Come, Lord Jesus, come."

Tom's brain tumor had taken from him all that his body had enjoyed, yet his spirit was full. He hungered to be clothed with that which is immortal; he hungered to be clothed with life.

One of the most helpful things God has taught me in dealing with cancer and pain is that my body is not me— not the real me, at least. When this life is over and this body dies, I will yet live. Death has been conquered, and I have an eternal building which awaits me.

In a way, it is like drinking coffee out of a cup in the morning. Perhaps you have a favorite cup that someone has given you, but it is not the cup itself you're interested in when the first rays of sunshine peek over the horizon. The cup merely holds the longed for coffee which helps us begin the day.

When I began to separate my body from "me," I began to better understand the beauty of eternity. I literally dream about the day when we all, like Tom, will be unburdened and clothed.

We are clay in the Potter's hand, and we are His to do with as He wills: "We have this treasure in jars of clay to show that this all-surpassing power is from God and not from us. We are hard pressed on every side, but not crushed; perplexed, but not in despair; persecuted, but not abandoned; struck down, but not destroyed" (2 Cor. 4:7-9).

No matter what happens to us in this world, God is at work, and He is the victor: "Therefore, we do not lose heart. Though outwardly we are wasting away, yet inwardly we are being renewed day by day" (2 Cor. 4:16).

Choose to see God's grace. Choose to be willing clay in the Potter's hands and to trust Him in the molding process. He knows what He is doing.

Questions to Consider

1. What are some of the struggles you thought were over which have recurred in your life? How are you handling those struggles?
2. What do you think it means for you to be "clay in the potter's hand?"
3. How do you want God to work in your life? What do you pray He will/will not do?
4. Do you understand what Paul means by "hard pressed, but not crushed; perplexed, but not in despair"? Talk about what those words mean in your own life.
5. If you were to go to the potter's house and look in the window as He works on the clay of your life, what would you see? What would He be smoothing? Refinishing? Remodeling? Preparing for the kiln?

10

Healing from the Inside Out

"The primal desire for fairness dies hard, and it should. Who among us does not sometimes yearn for more justice in this world here and now? Secretly, I admit, I yearn for a world 'fault-proof' against disappointment, a world where my magazine articles will always find acceptance and my body does not grow old and weak, a world where my sister-in-law does not deliver a brain-damaged child, and where Peggy Woodson lives into ripe old age. But if I stake my faith on such a fault-proof earth, my faith will let me down. Even the greatest of miracles do not resolve the problems of this earth: all people who find physical healing eventually die. . . . The cross of Christ may have overcome evil, but it did not overcome unfairness. For that, Easter is required. Someday God will restore all physical reality to its proper place under His reign. Until then, it is a good thing to remember that we live out our days on Easter Saturday."[1]

–Philip Yancey

Inadequate Solutions

People mean well when they give advice. They feel ruffled by our suffering and inadequate to help, so they offer whatever solution they imagine appropriate to the problem. Unfortunately, such efforts are at times clumsy and insensitive.

The age-old story of Job illustrates this situation well. His friends proved to be almost more exasperating than his loss or his illness.

When Job's friends first laid eyes on him, they gave him the best comfort they could—they sat silently with their friend for seven days and shared his tears. But then they began to offer unraveling advice. No longer did they bestow comfort, they gave opinions instead—opinions that held little consolation.

When North American Christians hear the word *suffering,* we immediately bristle. We are taught, from the time we are young, that life is in our back pocket. If we make the right choices and live morally, surely our lives will be relatively free from pain. Physical illness is a particularly troublesome problem that we imagine is meant for someone else.

When word got out about my cancer, I was immediately inundated with all kinds of advice about cures and treatments and spiritual cleansings. I heard the traditional message that I must be living in sin. I heard that my illness would go away if I had enough faith. I heard that it is not God's will for me to suffer. I heard that the only way to honor God is through physical healing. And I received numerous books and methods for conquering "The big C"—the dreaded disease that causes us all to quake in our boots.

I can tell you, from my own experience and that of many others I have known, that the promise or insistence on physical healing can be the heaviest burden a patient or a family member has to bear. Illness carries a weight of its own, without the added weight of thinking yourself responsible for the disease.

I will state right away that I fully believe in God's ability to heal the body. I believe that God can do anything in keeping with His character and nature. He has worked with my body and allowed me more days in this world, and for that privilege I am grateful.

The issue here is not whether God can heal. Instead, the issue rests on several questions. First, is physical healing promised in the atonement? Second, is God obligated to heal the physical diseases of believers when they have met certain conditions? Third, are miracles God's solution to man's problems?

I would like to address the basic issues these questions raise so that those who suffer need not bear a spiritual burden of this world's making. I would like to offer a perspective which may encourage those who are suffering as I have suffered.

Physical Healing Promised in the Atonement

If physical healing is promised in the atonement, why do all men and women die, and most from some kind of physical disease?

Since the beginning of time as we know it, only two people have avoided physical death altogether. Elijah and Enoch (some would add Melchizedek) were taken to meet the Lord without walking through the valley of the shadow. Aside from these men, however, all of us die—Christians and non-Christians, good and evil, spiritual and carnal, young and old.

Faced with such an obvious scenario, some say God-fearing believers do not die of illness, merely of accident or old age. The truth is, heart disease, kidney failure, and the disintegration of the body are illnesses in their own right. Whether we like it or not, we live in a diseased world, and our bodies are subject to this world's decay.

The Atonement question is addressed in a variety of biblical passages, but two particular passages are most often cited. The first passage is found in Chapter 53 of Isaiah (and its corresponding passage in Matthew 8:16-17), and the second in Psalm 103.

> Surely He took up our infirmities and carried our sorrows, yet we considered Him stricken by God, smitten by Him, and afflicted. But He was pierced for our transgressions, He was crushed for our iniquities; the punishment that brought us peace was upon Him, and by His wounds we are healed. We all, like sheep, have gone astray, each of us has turned to his own way; and the Lord has laid on Him the iniquity of us all (Isa. 53:4-6).

Every theologian or student of the Word has heard the arguments which exist over both the Hebrew and Greek words for *diseases, infirmities, afflictions,* and *healing,* so I won't try to deal with that which can easily be researched. I will, instead, speak candidly about my understanding of these verses as we attempt to consider the whole of God's Word and what we know to be true about His character.

Let me first point out that the Isaiah passage hinges on Christ's supremacy over sin. We would not have disease or any other problem were it not for the effect sin has had upon the world, beginning with Adam and Eve. Our problem is spiritual, not physical. Our problem is sin.

What we learn from this passage is that Christ took our sin and the penalty for that sin upon Himself. By doing this, He has freed us from the sentence of eternal death and brought us, instead, into life.

When we accept the sacrifice of Christ as our own, we have peace, and we are no longer slaves to sin. Nothing can steal that assurance from us. Nothing is more miraculous than this gift of redemption.

The fact that He took our sins upon Himself on the cross, however, does not free us from temptation and sin. While we live in this world in these bodies, we sin. We see this struggle all around us. How many ministers have succumbed to the desires of the body or to the pressures of a fishbowl existence? How many husbands have betrayed their wives? How many wives have forgotten to love and honor their husbands? How many churches have been split apart by the pride and jealousy which so easily entangle us?

How many of us lie to protect ourselves from consequences? How many of us covet that which belongs to someone else? How many of us hide our sins so that no one will know the weaknesses? How many of us are too engrossed in our own plans to be aware of the needs of others?

Phillip Yancey writes: "You don't have to look far—the church in Corinth, racism in South Africa, bloodshed in Northern Ireland, scandals among U.S. Christians—for proof that the church does not live up to God's ideal."[2]

We are free from sin's grotesque bondage and from its eternal darkness, but we are not, as yet, free from the everyday sins which plague our relationships and our lives. We would all like to cease from sin completely, but such a transformation still awaits us.

The same principle applies to physical illness. In Christ we are free from the eternal effects of such an illness, but we are not free from feeling its effects in this world. Cancer can only harm my body, it can do nothing to my soul. In fact, I will tell you that my soul has actually been enriched through facing this disease. We have a Saviour who creatively takes our times of suffering and works them together for good.

The atonement promises that those who accept Christ's sacrifice will no longer be bound by sin and its penalty, and it promises a resurrected body—free from sin, illness, and death. We do not yet have that resurrected body.[3] It is part of our hope—part of the future fulfillment of God's promise to His children.

> Praise the Lord, O my soul; all my inmost being, praise His holy name. Praise the Lord, O my soul, and forget not all His benefits—who forgives all your sins and heals all your diseases, who redeems your life from the pit and crowns you with love and compassion, who satisfies your desires with good things so that your youth is renewed like the eagle's (Ps. 103:1-5).

This passage reminds us that our Lord does indeed heal all our diseases, just as He forgives all our sin, but these verses do not tell us when and where such complete healing will take place.

David spoke of our sins being separated from us as far as the east is from the west (Ps. 103:12), and yet several of his psalms are prayers of repentance (Ps. 51; Ps. 130). He wept over the sins that plagued him as he sought to serve the Lord. If David had believed we no longer sin, he would not have needed to petition God for forgiveness. David knew God's cleansing power, but he also struggled with personal sin.

God cares about us individually, and He cares about a hurting and dying world. He does not promise, through the Atonement, to remove us from this world. He promises, instead, that we are more than conquerors (Rom. 8:35-37), both in this world and the next. We need not fear the process, for God is in control.

Is God Obligated to Provide Physical Healing?

Most believers would say that God is certainly not obligated to do anything other than that which He has covenanted to do. While we may agree on this point, we act, at times, as if He is obligated to do what we desire.

Those who believe that God is obligated to physically

heal us when we do the "right" things to bring about that healing usually cite passages like James 5 and Matthew 21, referring to Jesus' ministry of healing while He walked on this earth.

> Is any one of you in trouble? He should pray. Is anyone happy? Let him sing songs of praise. Is any one of you sick? He should call the elders of the church to pray over him and anoint him with oil in the name of the Lord. And the prayer offered in faith will make the sick person well; the Lord will raise him up. If he has sinned, he will be forgiven. Therefore confess your sins to each other and pray for each other so that you may be healed. The prayer of a righteous man is powerful and effective (James 5:13-16).

> I tell you the truth, if you have faith and do not doubt, not only can you do what was done to the fig tree, but also you can say to this mountain, 'Go throw yourself into the sea,' and it will be done. If you believe, you will receive whatever you ask for in prayer (Matt. 21:21-22).

Being physically ill is a frightening thing, particularly when your body is ravaged by some intruder who leaves behind pain, tremendous inconvenience, and, ultimately, unfair separation. We can't help but wish, at one time or another, that God would remove that intruder once and for all and leave us intact to continue our life.

We all want to believe that God will remove the unwanted and destroy that which threatens our security. Yet, we must realize that we cannot use His promises to demand that He comply with our own wishes. If we could, we would have all discovered long ago how to obtain everything on our list of "necessities."

The whole point of maturity is that we begin to want what God wants. We are not given freedom in order to serve our own desires, as Paul makes clear to the church in Galatia (Gal. 5:1-15), but in order to serve others in love. We must remember the example of our Lord: "Not My will, but Yours be done" (Luke 22:42).

The goal of maturity lies in being conformed to the image of Him whose name we bear. We have been given fair warning that part of the process includes suffering of different types and intensities. I find it a bit amusing when people say that it isn't God's will for me to suffer. First of all, if it isn't God's will for me to suffer and I am indeed suffering, then God is out of control, and we are all in big trouble.

Second, and most important, Jesus Himself told us that life would be difficult, not easy. He promised that we would have tribulation and grief and pain. He said we would be recipients of hatred and gossip and temptation and loss. The good news isn't that life in this world is perfect, it is that Jesus has overcome evil eternally, once and for all. When we suffer, it is no longer a deadend.

I have learned to pray differently since my illness. I used to tell God what I was sure He would agree with and ask Him to follow through on my request. I now tell Him what I am feeling and what I desire, yet I also make clear that I long for His will, not my own. I am borrowing that prayer, you will recall, and not from an unworthy source (Luke 22:42; John 12:27).

I didn't want to believe that God had cancer in mind for me, and you might argue that He does not will this to be happening in my life. But the fact is, it *is* happening. And I don't believe that anything occurs outside of God's sovereign will or His loving purpose. There is reason for our pain, hard as it is to see at times. There is design to our suffering and intention for our deaths. We prefer to be in charge of our own destiny, but God commands that control.

There is no magic formula which, when put together properly, yields healing. Those who try to link the miracle of healing to the faith of the one who is ill are only recognizing part of the truth.

Jesus healed in response to the faith of the afflicted one (Mark 5:34), and He healed in response to the faith of dedicated friends (Mark 2:5). But Jesus also healed those who were unable to exhibit faith (Mark 5:41-42), and He healed those who did not care for His miracles (John 5:1-15).

Jesus healed the "good" and He healed the "not-so-good." He healed believers and nonbelievers. He healed people with much faith and people with only a little, and He even healed bodies without healing souls. Jesus also brought the dead back to life when no one thought it possible.

There is no magic formula for healing, and such an expectation or implication can heap guilt and great disappointment on individuals or family members who are already suffering from their loss. It is not wrong to desire healing, but it is very shortsighted to insist that God always heals the body in this world.

I worked with a family several years ago that I will never forget. Their youngest child was ill with leukemia, and the parents were convinced that God would heal her. Though she grew progressively worse, they would not allow anyone to visit her who might cause her to doubt the healing they knew was certain.

She died. And the tragedy of her death was its aloneness. She left this world without the privilege of sharing her journey, and without the support of loving friends. Though I understand the parents' fear, I have often wondered who was the healthy one in that family.

Faith does not demand God's compliance with our wishes; faith holds onto the One who is true and onto His eternal promises. Faith the size of a mustard seed is faith enough for the healing. We need to trust God in our circumstances and not allow our faith to depend on today's physical relief.

I smile when people, disappointed that I am ill, pledge their prayers for my healing. You see, I believe that I am already healed in the manner that is eternally important. And I believe that my ultimate healing will be when I leave this body and go home.

To me, the true miracle is what God has done as He triumphed over evil with sacrifice and love. And He is performing a miracle within me. He is molding me into one who bears His image and sees through His eyes.

I know now that God knows best. And I know that His best for me is the only thing I really want. I have wept to think that pain and suffering are so feared, when the end result is knowing the One who died on the cross for our pardon.

Miracles . . . God's Solution?

The discussion of the third question falls naturally on the heels of what we have already discussed: Are miracles God's solution to man's problems?

I think back to my first few weeks of illness with great fondness. I had several people pray for my healing, and I was anointed with oil on more than one occasion. I have often wondered how I would have responded had God chosen to replace my missing ribs and free me from a body of illness.

I imagine I would have thrown a great party—a praise gathering—so that we could all thank God for the victory. And I am certain that such a miracle would have deepened my faith. But I also would not be the me I am today, and that is a sobering thought.

Through my cancer, God has shown me lessons about Himself and about love and frailty that I had never known before. Through my cancer, God has taught me about compassion and given me numerous opportunities to express that compassion to people in their pain.

I've learned about true healing, from the inside out. I've

118

spent more time loving God and others than I ever spent before my illness. I've learned to depend on God. I know what it means to rely on Him for literally all of my strength and ability.

Would I have learned those lessons with the same intensity or so early in life had I not been given the privilege of suffering?

Jesus did many miracles during His time on this earth. Sadly, we tend to look at the miracles and forget their purpose and their meaning. Jesus did not use miracles as the solution to problems. He used miracles to introduce Himself and His deity to the Jews and to this world.

One of the most troubling incidents in Scripture occurs right after the feeding of the 5,000. John records that Jesus fed the crowd and then joined His disciples at night on the other side of the lake. When the crowd noticed His disappearance, they too crossed to Capernaum in search of the One who had filled their stomachs.

> When they found him on the other side of the lake, they asked him, "Rabbi, when did You get here?"

> Jesus answered, "I tell you the truth, you are looking for Me, not because you saw miraculous signs, but because you ate the loaves and had your fill. Do not work for food that spoils, but for food that endures to eternal life, which the Son of Man will give you" (John 6:25-27).

The people wanted full stomachs again. They wanted their needs to be met effortlessly and on a regular basis. They were interested, not in the doer of the miracle, but in the benefit they derived.

If we are not careful, we will look to miracles with the same longing as those who were fed by five loaves and two fish. We will view miracles as solutions to our problems, rather than signs to point us to Christ.

Jesus wanted the people to respond to the miracles by coming to Him. When He saw what they demanded, He immediately moved the discussion to a deeper level:

> I am the Bread of Life. He who comes to Me will never go hungry, and he who believes in Me will never be thirsty. But as I told you, you have seen Me and still you do not believe (John 6:35-36).

The people grumbled and looked confused. But as Christians, we read those words and know exactly what they mean.

Jesus was not promising that we will never have to eat dinner or drink water again in this world. We do not take those words literally in the realm of the physical. The words are literal, all right, but in the eternal and spiritual sense. Jesus is the bread of life, and we must eat of His flesh and drink His blood. It is a hard teaching, and one that we only begin to comprehend.

Once we are believers, we no longer need miracles to draw us to the Lord. What we need is maturity and faithfulness and obedience and understanding. Miracles are not God's way of solving our problems; such a solution rests in our daily walk with Him.

We certainly do not have to look for suffering, but when it comes, we do not need to look to the miraculous to remove the suffering from our midst. God matures us through the difficulties of this world.

The miraculous is easy for God—He is Lord of all. But perhaps He knows that the path of suffering holds exactly what we need to be mature and complete, not lacking anything (James 1:4).

I was speaking for a conference one summer and was scheduled to begin the first session after a banquet and awards dinner. Just before the session began, a pastor introduced himself to me and said that he'd never seen a person who exhibited more joy. I smiled and thanked him for the encouragement, and we began to talk.

When he learned about my cancer, he asked what I was doing about the illness. I began telling him the course of treatment, which for me has been routine scans and blood tests, when he interrupted me with, "No, I mean what are you *doing* about it?"

Having met many who think I should be physically healed, I recognized where the conversation was going, and I reminded him that he had seen the joy that God has placed in my life. Then I asked him, "Doesn't such joy give testimony to the overwhelming power of God? Do we need physical miracles to praise Him or to see His handiwork?"

God's answer to our problems isn't always the miraculous—at least not the miraculous that we imagine. I see His working in my life as a very great miracle. I thank God every day that He did not remove my pain in October of 1982, for I have grown in ways I could never have imagined.

A Memorable Moment

In January of 1987, I boarded a train in Poland with seventeen young adults by my side. We had just completed a conference where we had shared about God's grace in our lives.

It was snowing very hard that day, and we were cold. A window in the train car was broken so that snow drifted in as we pulled out of the station. It would be a long and uncomfortable trip.

As the train chugged down the tracks, I heard a voice begin to sing God's praise. The tune was infectious. For the next few hours, we sang together and rejoiced in the Lord for all that He had done. Before we knew it, no one was giving thought to the cold or to the long journey that lay ahead of us.

As I gazed out the broken window, mountains and valleys, homes and steeples passed by, and so did my life. All I could think of that day was God's grace:

> *Thank You, Father, for all You have done in my life. Thank You for the pain and the illness and the faith that has brought me here to these people and to their love.*
>
> *Thank You for binding us together in the suffering that is common to man. Thank You that I am here, right now, cold and all.*
>
> *I know it may sound crazy, but since You already know, thank You for my loss. If I had to do this life all over, I'd choose this path again. You've loved me well.*

Questions to Consider

1. Is it all right for God not to heal physically?
2. Can you see how He uses even death or physical illness to bring glory to Himself?
3. What frightens you most about admitting that God might not always bring physical relief?
4. What have you learned about God in those moments when you experienced no immediate removal of pain?
5. Write your own psalm which expresses how the atonement benefits you today. What are the benefits that are still to come?

11

The Good Gifts of God

"Many of you reading this have experienced situations that did not make it or remain still unresolved. I simply invite you to remember the promise, 'surely goodness and mercy shall follow me all the days of my life.' The hound of heaven will pursue us recklessly until he can overwhelm us with his mercy, his love, and his goodness." [1]

—Tim Hansel

Calm in the Midst of Storm

When I first contracted cancer, so many questions came to mind: What was God doing? Was the diagnosis a mistake? Had I done something wrong? Was I supposed to see the cancer as a "good gift" from God?

Anytime we are confronted with suffering, the questions flow. And we are left with so few answers. We have to rely, instead, on faith and on what we know to be true about God.

In my own search for answers, I have found great comfort in one particular aspect of God's character: His goodness. When my pain seems impossible to bear, the thought of God's goodness soothes my distress like a calm in the midst of a storm. His goodness reminds me of the deeper waters to which He promises to guide me.

If we believe God is good, then all that He does and allows and accomplishes and plans in our lives must be in keeping with that goodness. Our only dilemma in this scenario becomes grasping the personal application of God's goodness and waiting patiently for its unfolding.

If, however, we believe that God is not entirely good or that His goodness is limited by some other force, then the suffering of this world falls under the whole new category of power. In this scenario, we must decide who is dishing out our pain and what he, she, or it is all about. We must also try to decipher if God has lost control, or if He is held captive by that which is troubling us.

I personally believe Scripture teaches that God is good. Goodness is His nature. And we all know that the white hat invariably beats the black hat in the end; those happy-ending movies are not unlike the real eternal thing.

I also believe that God gives good gifts to His children, that He works good in all things, and that His intentions are good. I believe God's goodness is all encompassing and that it gives us confidence as we seek to understand the suffering in life.

I have already used my own circumstances to illustrate what I believe to be true about God and His plan. I see both my suffering and the outcome of that suffering as part of God's goodness. I have watched His goodness spread through my life, over and over again. And I have literally seen God take the pain and mold it into something good, right before my eyes. My faith tells me that such transformation will continue.

God Is Good

Goodness begins with God because God is good. Jesus Himself attested to that fact as He conversed with the rich young man in Mark 10. "No one is good—except God alone" Jesus told him (Mark 10:18). And certainly Jesus would know.

The Greek word that describes God's goodness is a word that literally means, "that which, being good in its character or constitution, is beneficial in its effect."[2] That definition alone takes into consideration not only God's intrinsic goodness but also the outcome of that goodness. We can understand, then, why Jesus said that no one is good except God. The Creator of the universe is, Himself, both the cause and the effect of good.

The simplest of illustrations emphasizes this point. In the Texas springtime, few things are more beautiful than the blooming azalea bushes: white, pink, coral, and deep rose. Every year, as the cold of winter gives way to the warmth of spring, I discover that my azalea bushes are surrounded by tiny seedlings from an elm tree. The problem is, I don't have an elm tree in my yard! Can the azalea produce an elm? No. Instead, the wind carries the tiny seeds of the elm tree from someone else's yard and deposits those seeds among the other life in my garden. I am not even aware of the elm seedlings in my garden until they peek out from the soil in spring.

God is, Himself, good. We can get good from no other source, and the fruit of His labor must be good. Though another essence may plant its seed, nothing can destroy or deface the goodness of God.

Once we begin to understand God's goodness, we can begin to understand His good gifts. "Give thanks to the Lord Almighty, for the Lord is good; His love endures forever" (Jer. 33:11).

God's Good Gifts

During my illness I don't recall doubting the goodness of God, but I do recall questioning His commitment to give good gifts to His children. I had in mind my own list of good gifts, and cancer was not on that list.

Some who are struggling begin to doubt God's love. Some doubt their own ability to be loved. Some are certain that God must be punishing them for some unconfessed sin or dark secret. Suffering can cause those doubts, for we feel both angry and afraid, unsure and alone. The struggles of pain dig into the very depths of a person's faith in God, and search those depths for a little something called "hope."

In the Book of Genesis we read about a man named Joseph. He was the product of jealousy and bitterness, and he suffered under the hand of the same. His life was characterized by loss, yet he believed God gives good gifts.

Joseph was born into a very unhappy family. Jacob, Joseph's father, had two wives who were sisters. Jacob had worked seven years for the privilege of marrying Rachel, the younger daughter of Laban. He was in love with her and wanted her as his wife, but Laban had something different in mind.

The wedding was grand. Both wine and good food flowed well into the morning, and I assume Jacob drank until his awareness was dulled. Though it's hard to imagine such carelessness, Jacob awoke the next morning to find himself partnered to the older daughter, Leah. Jacob was furious, but by law he could do nothing. And so Jacob worked another seven years for the bride of his dreams, Rachel. It is this deceit that leads to the birth of Joseph and his brothers.

God knew that Jacob loved Rachel rather than Leah, so we are told that God opened Leah's womb and closed Rachel's. So began the war between an unloved sister and an infertile one.

Ten children were born in the course of the next few years—some to Leah, some to Rachel's servant, and others to Leah's servant. Every child bore the name of the mothers' frenzy, and every child bore the weight of the battle (Gen. 29:31–30:24).

Leah was sure that each new boy would enable her to buy her husband's love. And Rachel was determined to keep her sister from enjoying the fruit of her womb. Day after day, child after child, they battled for the love of one man.

It is no wonder that when Rachel finally bore Jacob a son, another round of hatred began. This time, the jealousy raged, not only between the two sisters, but also between the children. Rachel named her son Joseph, and he was well-loved. He even wore a coat of many colors which his father made specifically for him. And so the other brothers despised this one who grew up in their shadow.

Genesis 37 records that young Joseph, then seventeen, began to dream dreams and relate them to the family. The dreams seemed arrogant to the brothers, so they were only too anxious to remove this burr under the saddle of their lives.

One day, Joseph was sent to see if all was well with his brothers in the field. At the time he was not aware of their desire to kill him, but their sentiments became clear when he arrived. The ten threw their brother into an empty cistern while they ate lunch and considered their options.

I picture Joseph only a few feet from the brothers as they ate. I wonder how he felt as he heard them plotting to end his life. Did he pray that their anger would subside? Had he known how much they hated him?

After some discussion, the brothers decided to sell Joseph rather than kill him. "After all," one of them said, "he is our brother, our own flesh and blood" (Gen. 37:27).

I doubt if that made Joseph feel any better. Joseph was sold, that day, into slavery. And as if that were not enough, his robe was taken by his brothers, torn in two, and dipped in blood. The plan was to tell their father Jacob that a wild animal had devoured his precious son. And so the plan was dutifully executed, and the object of their jealousy was disposed of—or so they thought.

Years went by, and Jacob never fully recovered from losing his son. I have wondered, many times, just what the brothers did to lessen their guilt. Did they feel more loved with Joseph out of the way? Probably not. Were they able to forget their deed? I doubt it.

And poor Joseph, what happened to him? Where was God when this young boy was victimized by his brothers? Why didn't God let the plan backfire or somehow notify Jacob that his son was still alive? Where was God when Joseph needed him most?

God gives good gifts to His children, but there are times when the gifts are hard to unwrap and even harder to accept. I can't imagine how lonely, betrayed, and insecure Joseph must have felt in the hands of the Egyptian slave traders.

In his new position, Joseph tried to do what was right. Still, it seemed that his pain was destined to increase. One day the wife of Joseph's employer tried to seduce the young slave. He resisted, but she only tried again a few days later. This time, he left his cloak in her hand as he fled, and she accused him of trying to rape her. Once again, Joseph was punished for doing what was right, and prison became his home.

Where was God this time? Wasn't the rejection of his family enough? Hadn't Joseph proved himself a godly man? Was there any purpose in this new accusation and punishment?

In the Book of Genesis, we read that "the Lord was with [Joseph]; He showed him kindness and granted him favor in the eyes of the prison warden. So the warden put Joseph in charge of all those held in the prison, and he was made responsible for all that was done there" (Gen. 39:21-22).

I wonder if Joseph understood God's kindness, or if he thanked God daily for His good gifts. This was not a short-term problem in Joseph's life, he had to trust God for years and against many odds.

As Philip Yancey puts it:

> If anyone had a valid reason to be disappointed in God, it was Joseph, whose valiant stabs at goodness brought him nothing but trouble . . . but shift, for a moment, to the perspective of God as parent. Had he deliberately "pulled back" to allow Joseph's faith to reach a new level of maturity? And could this be why Genesis devotes more space to Joseph than to any other person? Through all his trials, Joseph learned to trust: not that God would prevent hardship, but that He would redeem even the hardship.[3]

I do not pretend to understand God's gifts. There are times when it feels like what He allows isn't good at all. Certainly cancer or any kind of suffering feels anything but good at the time.

So how can we know God is good? How can we know He is giving the gifts that are best for us and for others?

If, as a parent, you could see into the future and know exactly what your child would need, would you not long to prepare him for future tasks or potential pain?

We see in a mirror dimly. We do not know what we will need tomorrow or the next day or in eternity. God *does* know, but He doesn't tell us all that is in His storehouse of information. He asks us to trust Him, and that is often difficult, at best.

Children have a hard time understanding why parents say no. And to a teenager, taking the car or staying out late or dating someone older seem so innocent, so appropriate for now. They are rarely concerned with tomorrow.

Parents, however, are coming from a different perspective. They understand a bit more about life and certainly about what can go wrong. Parenting isn't easy. Parents must try to do what is best for a child who may not agree.

Which of you, if his son asks for bread, will give

him a stone? Or if he asks for a fish, will give him a snake? If you, then, though you are evil, know how to give good gifts to your children, how much more will your Father in heaven give good gifts to those who ask Him? (Matt. 7:9-11)

God is good, and so are the gifts He gives. They may not look too appetizing today, but tomorrow will reveal the reason for the menu. God comes from the realm of eternity, and He is preparing us for the same.

God Works Good

One of the first verses I memorized as a child was Romans 8:28: "And we know that in all things God works for the good of those who love Him, who have been called according to His purpose."

The words sounded nice, but as a child I had no idea of their relevance or the comfort that they would one day provide. I also didn't memorize the verses that follow: "For those God foreknew He also predestined to be conformed to the likeness of His Son, that He might be the firstborn among many brothers. And those He predestined, He also called; those He called, He also justified; those He justified, He also glorified" (Rom. 8:29-30).

The words of that passage give us more information about the working out of God's good gifts than we can fully grasp. Most of us desire comfortable gifts from God, but He is not in the business of making us feel good today. As these verses remind us, God cares most about who we are becoming and what we need in order to be conformed to the likeness of His Son.

Research has proven that children who live in homes where there is little care for the future are in a very disadvantaged position. The parent whose only burden is getting through today with the least possible struggle produces a child who has little concern with his or her tomorrow.

Like a concerned parent, God is in the business of whole-person development. He is not as concerned with our comfort today as He is with our character tomorrow.

God sent His Son into this world with our future in mind. The process was started on the cross, but it continues today. We are daily being made into the likeness of Him who has gone before us. We are predestined, called, justified, and glorified; and, if you'll recall, the glorification of Jesus included the greatest moment of human suffering ever known.

All of our lives hold purpose in suffering. Paul was prevented from going to Spain and held in house arrest, yet many came to Christ as a result of his ordeal. Even those in Caesar's household were introduced to the Gospel (Phil. 1:13; 4:22).

Stephen was martyred for his firm belief in God, yet his life ended in triumph and tribute to His Saviour. Before the last stone fell, every person present heard the testimony of Christ's death and resurrection. It was that testimony which would later be instrumental in turning Saul to Paul (Acts 7:54–8:1; 9:1-19).

Daniel lived in captivity for years, and faced test after test of his faith. God never left the prophet alone, even for a moment. Daniel was given truths about the future that all of us long to behold—and all in the midst of his imprisonment (see the Book of Daniel).

Life is painful, but God is bigger than the pain. And God has in mind our completion. "The Lord will fulfill His purpose for me" David stated. "Your love, O Lord, endures forever—do not abandon the works of Your hands" (Ps. 138:8). The psalmist knew that God could not abandon those who are "fearfully and wonderfully made" (Ps. 139:14).

Joseph knew that the Lord had a purpose for him. He also knew that in all things God had been working for his good and would complete that good. I don't know how this young man discovered such Truth, but it was clear that he knew the Truth and that his trust was in God.

After Joseph had spent years in prison, Pharaoh sent for the young man to interpret a dream. Joseph interpreted the dream to mean there would be seven years of plenty followed by seven years of terrible famine.

Pharaoh began to prepare for this coming famine, and he needed the wisest and most discerning man possible to lead the country through the coming devastation. He chose Joseph.

Those years Joseph had spent in prison, the pain that he had endured at the hands of his brothers, and the faithful service he had exhibited all had a purpose. They taught Joseph obedience and prudence and long-suffering and character, and that is exactly what God needed in the man who would lead the Egyptians through the famine.

Joseph was thirty years old when he was put in charge, and he did exactly what he had been prepared to do. He stored the grain, readied the country, and enjoyed personal success. He even named his children after his new prosperity:

> Joseph named his firstborn Manasseh and said, "It is because God has made me forget all my trouble and all my father's household." The second son he named Ephraim and said, "It is because God has made me fruitful in the land of my suffering" (Gen. 41:51-52).

When famine came, Joseph's brothers were sent to Egypt to get food for the family. They had no idea that Joseph was in charge; they had no idea that Joseph was even alive. In fact, they didn't even recognize their long lost brother.

Though his pain was great, Joseph finally revealed his identity to the brothers. They quaked in their boots. They expected terrible retribution, but Joseph's response was wise and loving and very insightful. "Do not be distressed and do not be angry with yourselves for selling me here, because it was to save lives that God sent me ahead of you" (Gen. 45:5).

Was Joseph slightly crazy? Had the time in prison affected his memory? No, he just believed that God is in control, and that He is working, in all things, for the good of those who love Him.

My cancer is no different than Joseph's abandonment, nor than the disappointments of countless others throughout history. Suffering comes in all shapes and sizes, but it is still suffering.

God is working in my life, and He is working in yours. The only thing that we must do is believe God. God is good, He gives good gifts, and He is committed to working in all things for our good. It is as if God is sewing together each thread of our lives into an exquisite tapestry of good.

Intentions of Good

One of the hardest concepts to grasp is God's ability to see us, not in time, but outside of time. It is we who measure in seconds, minutes, hours, and years; but God does not measure that way, nor does He see us through "time-colored glasses."

God sees who we were, who we are, who we will become—and all at the same time. "A day is like a thousand years, and a thousand years like a day," wrote Peter (2 Peter 3:8). Perhaps he was trying to teach us to free God from our measurement.

Joseph was taken away from his family at seventeen. By thirty, he was finally released from prison and allowed to use his good gifts. Thirteen years was a long time for the young man to hold on to hope; yet to God, the time that it took to prepare Joseph, his brothers, and the world was no time at all!

No matter what happens to us—whether we become ill, lose someone we love, suffer the emotional pain of separation, or countless other possibilities, God is at work. And

His intentions of good have long been laid as the framework for the events of this world.

When Satan approached God for permission to bother Job, God already had control of the final outcome. God is good, and the outcome of any event will always be to His glory. All Satan actually did was strengthen God's servant, and that was fine with God.

When Satan provided a banquet table of temptations for Jesus, the temptations only strengthened our Lord and provided a way for Jesus to understand our troubles. Satan was used to accomplish God's good.

God is a planner. He has intentions. He knows where He is going and how to accomplish exactly what He desires to accomplish. Because He is good, His intentions are good, and we can count on that in our own lives.

Joseph's brothers were completely startled when Joseph revealed his identity. I imagine that each one looked around the room for a way of escape. It must have been the most uncomfortable day of their lives.

After introductions, the plan was laid to reunite Jacob with his beloved son. Joseph wept with his brothers and he kissed them. I can imagine the conversation as they left their brother's presence that day.

"What are we going to tell our father? How will we explain that coat—and the blood? Will our father remove our blessings? Do we trust Joseph's kiss? Do you think he's going to harm us? Why in the world did we ever come to Egypt in the first place?"

The brothers did not know what to think, because they were judging their brother by their own behavior and schemes. They had sold him in anger and forgotten him, now he was offering to care for them. They couldn't comprehend the forgiveness.

Jacob was reunited with his son, and Joseph indeed took care of them all, but the brothers continued to nurture a seed of distrust toward Joseph. We see that seed sprout at the end of the story.

When Joseph's brothers saw that their father was dead, they said, "What if Joseph holds a grudge against us and pays us back for all the wrongs we did to him?" (Gen. 50:15)

Scripture records that Joseph wept over his brothers' suspicion. Then he spoke words that ring loud with faith and truth.

Don't be afraid. Am I in the place of God? You intended to harm me, but God intended it for good to accomplish what is now being done, the saving of many lives. So then, don't be afraid. I will provide for you and your children (Gen. 50:19-21).

The world is full of evil, physical death, and weakness. Divorce, painful separation, and hatred come in all shapes and sizes. Starvation and war abound, as do famine and disaster. Our world is full of hostile and greedy people—those who lie, deceive, destroy, and plan the most devious of deeds.

But above all of these, there is God. No matter what pain or suffering the world dishes out, the Master has intended good in all things.

The purpose which God has given me in my suffering is far more encompassing than I had imagined. In fact, I am certain I will not comprehend its breadth until eternity, and maybe not even then. God has used me to be a conduit of His comfort, and that alone makes the pain worthwhile.

I have talked to many believers in deep pain. Some become angry and bitter, some refuse to accept the circumstances, some see themselves as cursed or useless. Some keep muttering that "life is unfair." I have found that no matter how much Scripture they read or how much encouragement they receive, some people do not want to see suffering from God's perspective. It is tragic.

On the other hand, every believer who sees himself or herself as a blessed child of a loving Father cannot mistake God's goodness. Even in their pain, such people reflect more joy and meaning than most of us show in a lifetime.

The definition of good is the definition of God. He is "that which, being good in its character or constitution, is beneficial in its effect." God is the cherry tree of goodness, the cause and the effect! And we are both the recipients and the players in the working out of that good.

God is good. God gives good gifts. God works good in all things. And God's intentions are good. Joseph learned the truth that set him free—even in a world of darkness— and we can do the same.

Questions to Consider

1. What does God's goodness have to do with your pain right now?
2. Chart your life. On a time line note significant dates and experiences which have had an effect on your life. Include both the painful periods and the easier times.
3. What can you learn from your chart about God's purposes in your life? About your response to God?
4. Have there been times when your suffering has proved to be a blessing, in some way, to someone else? If so, when and how?
5. What do you think helped Joseph to accept the events of his life as part of God's goodness? How can Joseph's awarenesses help you?

12

To Friends and Family

"*People sometimes ask what impact the accident had on my family. It has been extensive. Statistics show that trauma of any sort will have a major influence on a family's survival. It took me years to understand that my pain was often worse on my family and my friends than it was on me. For a long period of time, my selfish preoccupation simply blinded me to that fact.*"[1]

–Tim Hansel

For Better or for Worse

I believe that the family and friends of one who is in pain suffer the most. Particularly when the suffering comes in the form of a physical problem, those closest to the afflicted one have a very difficult road to walk. Those who are watching must do a great deal of trusting and loving when they would just as soon be doing. It is difficult to know how to help.

When we first found out about my cancer, my mother and father were stunned. Here they were at the end of life, so to speak, yet a cruel twist of events was threatening to take their daughter's life first. Children only barely prepare themselves for their parents to die, but parents almost never prepare for the death of their child.

Helpless is the most common word I hear in the discussions I have with family members and friends of those who are suffering. Our whole society is very remedy oriented, and so we find it excruciatingly difficult to sit back while some enemy haunts the one we love.

Many people have expressed to me the wish that they could bear the suffering for their loved one, and I understand. My good friend and partner in ministry has stood by for years and watched me struggle. There are days I know he would rather bear the pain himself than watch me cry, but such an arrangement is impossible.

What can a parent do? What can a child do? What can a sister or a brother do? And what can a friend do to lessen the severity of the pain in the life of the beloved?

A Delicate Balance

Jesus had a marvelous skill. He could help bear people's burdens without taking responsibility for their entire load. Even in paying for our sin, He took the eternal burden, yet left us with individual responsibility. It is important for us to discover and practice this balance.

One day, while Jesus and the disciples were walking, a blind man caught our Lord's attention, and Jesus took pity on him (John 9). He made mud with His saliva and then placed that mud in the man's sightless eyes. On the surface, Jesus' action seemed thoughtless.

You know the next part of the story. The man went to wash in the Pool of Siloam, and then he could see! Unfortunately, the Pharisees were not too happy with that miracle, and they began to taunt and question the man about the One who brought healing.

When the blind man seemed to need Jesus the most, the Teacher could not be found. Why would the miracle worker heal the man and then disappear?

The unfolding of the story seems to fill in those missing gaps. Jesus wanted the man to stand on his own two feet and choose to believe even when the Pharisees scorned and accused him. At last, when the man had maintained his position and stood alone once more, Jesus appeared to him and welcomed him into the kingdom. Our Lord took part of the man's burden, but not the entire load.

The tendency of family and friends is to grab the whole load, as if they can be responsible without rest or limit. As you can imagine, that is why the energy of the family often gives out before the death or healing of the suffering individual.

If we accept the entire load, we stand in the way of God's doing in the sufferer the work that He desires. It is crucial that we encourage the afflicted one to accept and continue accepting his or her own cross.

Burden-bearing must be kept in balance so that both care-givers and patients can embrace what God wants to teach through the suffering.

To the Family and Friends

We've already explored the biblical value of bearing one another's loads. Let me offer, in the remaining pages of this chapter, a few practical suggestions to help guide you through the process.

Trust God
First, and foremost, TRUST GOD with your loved one, and I do not mean for that to sound trite.

God will give your husband or wife or child or mother or father or friend exactly what that person needs to cope with the suffering. I think one of the reasons that suffering and death are hardest on friends and family is precisely because we are forced to observe—we are not the one receiving special grace from God.

God gives all of us strength to deal with our difficulties, but the strength He gives is apportioned according to the need. A parent watching a child suffer is granted a different sort of grace than that which is given the child. An elderly parent who is ill is given a different sort of strength than that which the family receives.

God really does meet our need, and He will give your loved one just what is necessary to endure or to overcome, to live or to die. Trusting Him to do just that lessens the pressure on everyone. He *does* know what He is doing and why, even though His purposes often elude us.

Don't Try to Fix

Second, let me remind you that, while we often play the "I-can-fix-it" game, it is not our role in life to make everything OK for those around us. It is our privilege to care for those we love as best we can, but we must realize that it is not our job, nor is it within our control, to fix life for someone else.

This is a tough suggestion to follow. I can't tell you how many times I have seen the family and friends take over for the afflicted one and begin making all the decisions. They mean well at the time, but fixing becomes a burden to both parties.

Sometimes—oftentimes, life cannot be fixed. Keep that in mind, and don't equate loving with taking away the problem. Love the person in the midst of the problem. Such love will go far.

I have friends who try to fix my situation. They cut out articles or come up with ways that my problem can be solved. Their intentions are fine, but their actions make the situation more difficult for me. I want proper care, but I want a godly attitude even more. I am trying to learn from the problems as I go, and I am trying to trust God to lead me.

When we try to fix, we often lose sight of the fact that God is interested in something bigger than bringing immediate healing. In our suffering He wants to bring us to maturity in Him, and we need to help our loved ones take that step as well.

Be with the Sufferer

Third, it is important to just be with the person who is suffering. Sometimes a phone call or card is sufficient (particularly in long-distance relationships), but there is no substitute for simply "being with" one who is in pain. *You* are the very best gift you can give.

We saw how Jesus wanted the company of His three closest friends as He went to the mountain to pray one last time. His friends could do nothing to alter the situation—they could not fix our Lord's pain. Jesus simply wanted His friends close by while He prepared to carry His biggest load yet. How true it is that the company of the ones we love is a soothing balm to any soul.

When you are with me, you tell me that I am significant to you and that you are willing to be part of my experience. That action speaks a thousand words.

Bring a book and sit awhile. Stay and relax. Let the person who is struggling enjoy your presence and learn to enjoy his or her presence as well. It is healing just to have someone there.

Demonstrate Acceptance and Touch

Fourth, learn to accept and to touch. These are two simple actions, but their comfort is far from simple.

Since the day of my surgery back in 1982, I have had the great privilege of friends who are not afraid to touch or accept me in whatever state I happen to be for the day. I feel so much better when I know they care.

Acceptance and touch are two special ingredients in the handling of life's pains. Giving this gift to one who is suffering relieves much of that person's burden—it provides a kind of strength that can't be purchased, swallowed, or otherwise contrived.

When a person is physically or emotionally down, he or she is likely to feel unlovable or unworthy or untouchable. I think of that woman who reached out to touch the hem of Jesus' garment after having been untouchable herself for twelve long years. I can almost feel her joy when the touch proved to be full of love (Mark 5:21-34).

Jesus accepted the woman in her unclean state, and He received her touch. He didn't chide her for dirtying His cloak or delaying His important journey. She was important to Him, and He cared.

Inside every body is a creation of God—a creature who longs to be close to love. We don't feel as strange or separated when someone reaches out to touch what may be an unlovely body or a hurting soul.

If someone walks into the hospital room, stands far away, and speaks of things that seem meaningless to the world of the sufferer, the sharing between the two is limited. But if someone enters the hospital room and steps into the moment with warmth and acceptance, real comradery develops between the patient and the visitor.

Acceptance and touch are amazing gifts. They tell me that I am loved and heard and needed by someone in this world.

View Suffering as a Gift

Fifth, try to see the person who suffers as someone who is specifically gifted—not as someone to be pitied. When people see me as special and as a person with purpose, I have a much easier time seeing myself that way.

I remember my friend asking me each day in the hospital, "what are you learning?" While the first few days I had nothing to say, by the third day I was ready. I took pen and paper in hand and scribbled (very literally!), "Yesterday I thought I would live forever, but today I know I'm going to die." Those words contained no profound insight, but they helped me establish a pattern of expecting growth. My friend did not pity me, he saw me as a person who is important to God and His plan.

Try to encourage those of us who are suffering to grow. Try to draw us out of our shells of pity and fear. We need your help to see the learning that God has in store for us.

If you are doubting God's wisdom, it is hard for we who suffer to see His hand. We need you to believe that God gives good gifts to His children—even if they come in un-lovely packages.

Be Honest

Sixth, respect the one you love and deal honestly with that person. This is especially important when discussing major issues such as the nature of an illness or the quality of life that can be expected.

Honesty is also crucial in day-to-day conversations. For instance, it is fine to tell me that I look like I am in pain. If I am, the fact that you noticed will only serve to encourage me. If, on the other hand, every time we meet, you say I look great, I will begin to dread that part of the conversation. I don't have "permission" to feel bad or look bad if all you are able to say is that I look great.

I know it seems encouraging to speak only positive words, but I need to hear reality, and it helps me to open up if I know that you too are able to handle what is really going on.

People who are dying know they are dying. People who are depressed are also well aware of their condition. Avoiding the reality does little good, and often much harm. It is so much better to build on a foundation of trust.

Let me know what the doctors say, walk with me through my fears, tell me if you are struggling or need a break. Build and sustain our relationship on honesty.

Share Your Feelings

The seventh bit of advice is simple: don't be afraid to say what YOU feel. If you come to see me one day, and it makes you feel like crying to see me in pain, then please cry. I will count it real friendship to know that you care enough to openly express your feelings for me.

If you are finding my illness difficult to bear, then tell me. I know that sounds harsh, but it is very important. Let me know what *you* need, or we will lose the two-way nature of the relationship.

When you are afraid to be anything but fun, resourceful, and happy, I don't have the chance to see what you are really like or how my pain affects you. Such hiding also leaves you with a tremendous storehouse of unexpressed and unexplored emotions.

It is fine if you cry with me — for me or for yourself. I can feel a part of you much better that way. And it is fine if you are angry or tired or hurt or frustrated. Let me be part of your struggle.

There are those who say that the caregiver should not share his or her burdens with the one in pain. After all, we imagine the burden of the afflicted one to be heavy enough without our addition. That rationale sounds good, but it doesn't work.

The one who is suffering knows when something is wrong with family or friends. By expressing your concerns, you will save the sufferer from worrying unnecessarily about you. Let the one in pain in on your own load of suffering. Both your burdens will be so much lighter.

Be a Listener

Learn to be an active listener. In other words, participate in my reactions, thoughts, doubts, and questions. I know you have no answers — that is not what I expect or need. I just want a partner in the process.

I have dealt with several families whose greatest sorrow after the death of a loved one is that no one really talked to the person about the things he or she was thinking. Trying not to discourage the afflicted one, the family members and friends missed some great conversations.

Listening is an art, and a very welcome gift. Ask the sufferer how he or she is feeling and then listen for awhile. We tend to feel uncomfortable when there is "dead air." We often talk about meaningless things just to relieve the tension of no talk at all. Don't be afraid of "dead air," it is a nice sound in friendship.

Listen. Talk back. Feel in return. Be an active participant in the process.

Be Patient

Finally, be patient. Give me time, and know that I need you. Even though I may be silent or even distant at times, it is not because I don't want you around.

When the pain or the feelings of loss or the physical symptoms rob me of my usual joy, I may have little to say. I want you and need you, though, even if I can't always express that need.

Many family members or friends of a person who is suffering tell me that their loved one is angry or depressed and, therefore, can't talk about the problem. While talking may be difficult, that is not the real tragedy. The real tragedy is if the loved one quits trying to communicate because of a little resistance or a lot of emotion on the part of the sufferer.

Stay with me awhile! Encourage me by your presence, and I'll come around. It takes times to grow through and with the difficulties of this life. And if I am dying, I have so much to offer you as I walk through my last days on this earth.

As a Christian, I'm on my way home, and that is the culmination of joy and hope. I'd love to share the journey with you, if you have time.

Words of Encouragement

Let me simply remind you that suffering is a process. Whether it spans a long period of time or is limited in scope, it is a process. And as members of the body of Christ, suffering is a process that leads us into greater maturity and conformity to the image of Jesus Christ.

When life doles out pain, our immediate response is to halt the process or limit the extent of the casualty. We want to protect the ones we love, and we know of no better way than to fix the problem or carry the load ourselves.

I understand the dilemma, but the better way is to consider what we might do to aid one another in the process of maturity. We have nothing to fear and certainly nothing to lose. We are eternally the children of God. He knows what is best.

We all hope suffering will be unnecessary, especially as it applies to those we love—the young, the "good," the sincere. But I know now that we are privileged children of God for whom suffering and death are not enemies. Instead, they are appointed teachers of perseverance, character, and hope (Rom. 5:1-5). I, for one, have learned to be humbly grateful for the lessons.

We serve a God who does not make mistakes, and some of the experiences He allows us in this life include loss, suffering, and pain. Great men and women of Scripture learned eternal lessons from the very instructors we fear.

I know that it is far easier to quote a truth from Scripture than it is to live that truth. And I know that the truths I've shared often fail to soothe the grief of the family members and friends. I can only tell you that in my own life suffering has been a great gift which God has used to shower good things on me. I do not feel abandoned by my Lord or lost in a maze with no escape.

If we see the process of suffering as unacceptable, then we miss our opportunity to participate in the growth of those we love. If we shut ourselves off from the possibility of good emerging from the painful, then we put on dark glasses of impossibility and frustration.

Help those you love to see a bigger picture—one of a

loving God who longs to give good gifts to His children. He fed thousands through the pain of young Joseph. He rescued Caesar's household through the imprisonment of Paul. He allowed Job to see Him, though all of his earthly possessions were destroyed. And He offers us eternal life through the pain and death of His Son.

While the suggestions I've offered are general ones, I pray they will help you in your day-to-day dealing with someone who is suffering. What I am offering, really, are the basics of relationships—basics that we tend to forget when life is hard.

Don't say, "Those tips won't work" before you've tried them. And don't stop trying after one or two failures. It will take time for everyone involved to adjust to suffering.

Above all else, please don't underestimate what God is doing in you or in the ones you love. Expect growth. Expect His presence. Trust His judgment. And watch for the working out of His plan. There is a glorious rainbow at the end of the storm—that promise never fails. How marvelous to help someone else see the colors.

Questions to Consider

1. What are the most difficult things you must do as you watch your loved one suffer?
2. Write a letter to God about the suffering. Let Him know what you are really feeling and the questions that are in your mind. Writing will help you better understand what is going on inside of you.
3. If you were really ill yourself, or in pain, what do you think you would need or want from family and friends?
4. Which of the suggestions in this chapter do you find the most difficult to do? Why?
5. What do you need to do for your loved one today? Is there something left unsaid or undone that you can work on right now? Remember, if you haven't tried, you do not know what will happen.

13

To the Minister

"We dare not confine theology to seminary coffee shops where professors and students play mental badminton. It affects all of us. Some people lose their faith because of a sharp sense of disappointment with God. They expect God to act a certain way and God 'lets them down.' Others may not lose their faith, but they too experience a form of disappointment. They believe God will intervene, they pray for a miracle, and their prayers come back unanswered."[1]

–Philip Yancey

A Difficult Calling

The job of the minister is difficult any time, but it can be exceptionally stressful in a situation where intense suffering is involved. I have learned, through the years, that young ministers find this part of pastoring particularly difficult.

My first "ministry to ministers" came in the early months of my illness. I was asked to conduct a conference for pastors in which I shared the struggles and pains of terminal illness. I remember thinking my words would probably be of little value; after all, ministers see suffering every day. I was mistaken.

Each person at that conference knew the overwhelming feeling of helplessness when trying to comfort one who is suffering, and each person there was also well aware of just how empty biblical promises can seem in moments of deep loss. We had a great day of sharing what we felt and discussing what we longed to impart to people in their pain.

It isn't easy to meet the needs of the sick person as well as those of the family. In fact, trying to pastor in such situations is far more difficult than delivering any sermon. It is personal. Those who hurt are looking for personal assurance from the minister—and from God.

I have known the blessing of being ministered to in my own suffering. I have had the encouraging company of a man whose God is big enough to deal with even the most devastating troubles of this world. Such faith has spurred me on to capture this perspective, for there is nothing quite like a lift from one whose life rests in the hands of the Father.

I have also been privileged to minister to others in their pain. I am regularly called on to spend time with those who are suffering and to train caregivers in churches, hospitals, hospices, and other organizations.

I have worked with caregivers, and I have walked with sufferers through the valley of the shadow, and I do not regret the journey. My days have been enriched by accompanying others through disappointments and discoveries, and I would like to encourage you as you do the same.

As I see the situation, there are several things which you, the minister, can uniquely provide as you endeavor to respond to the deepest needs of God's children. I have divided the suggestions into two categories: truths to remember, and truths to convey. Let me briefly outline these thoughts for you in the hope of lightening your load.

Truths to Remember

As we look into some truths to remember, keep in mind that these truths are basic understandings about life and about people. There is nothing new here, except a quiet encouragement from someone who hurts.

There Is No Need to Fix

First of all, realize that it is not your job to alter circumstances. It *is* the minister's job to love and to reflect the brilliant nature of God in an otherwise bleak situation.

As pastor of God's sheep, it is difficult to stand by when a wolf sneaks in and threatens the flock's security. It is natural for you to want to guard and protect—to chase away the foe. Remember, however, that suffering is not a wolf in the life of the believer. It is, instead, one of the ways God uses to bring His sheep into maturity. Suffering then, is not a problem that needs to be fixed.

How helpless we feel when we can't control circumstances. I know. I face that dilemma every day of my life. I wish I could make it easier on my body, but I can't. We are all fixers, and fixers are frustrated when things don't get better.

As a minister, your job is not to change events or make the pain go away; your job is far more significant than that. Your task is to offer the gift of perspective, helping sufferers see God in the midst of their pain. It is God's purpose, His love, His comfort, and His perspective for which we hunger and thirst in the thick of a storm.

Although a family may seem helpless and greatly in need of someone to make it all OK, that is not your job. You are needed to draw them into the company of peace, hope, encouragement, and love.

The Importance of Honesty

Please write on your forehead that a suffering person needs honesty. You may be in for a battle to convince the family of this need, but the person who is hurting or dying needs to understand what is happening.

Those of us who know we are ill are not surprised when our suspicions are confirmed. Even though we may experience shock or fear or anger or resentment at the news, it is best to let us know what is taking place in our bodies. We know something is wrong, and we will adjust more quickly and more healthily if someone will help us face the facts.

I can candidly say that there are few things I find more tragic than watching someone die who has not had the chance to talk openly about death, pain, fear, love, and eternity. A person who is dying or facing chronic pain can offer us so much if we give that person the chance. Protection from reality is a terrible thing for a child of God to experience. Maturity comes with a progressive acceptance of what is. It does not come with denial or dishonesty.

Do not expect the patient, and least of all the family members, to respond courageously in the first stages of the pain. And please don't feel discouraged about your ministry if the sufferers are sad, depressed, or angry. In the long run, honesty pays off with healthy results. It takes time to adjust to the new game plan. The fact that you are there speaks louder than words. The family and the struggler will look to you for guidance, so lead them gently down the path of openness.

The Healing Power of Touch

Several days after my first surgery for cancer, I was visited by one of the pastors at a local church. I still remember that visit.

Stepping into the room, the pastor called to me and said, "How are you doing, Miss Chapin? We want you to know we're praying for you! Take care!" And off he went, back through the same door he had entered only moments before.

Though ministers rarely call out from the door of the

hospital room, perhaps this exaggerated example will serve to make a point. When you visit a person in pain, keep in mind that the gift of touch is a remarkable one.

People who are suffering often feel untouchable. They feel unattractive and, many times, embarrassed by their looks or by the myriad of tubes that keep them going when the body's ability wears thin.

Reaching out and offering your touch is like offering a soothing balm or a drink from a cool spring. Touch bridges the gaps of physical constraint and joins hearts. Touch can work miracles of love.

I was training pastors on this very topic one evening when I was asked, "What if I don't know the person? Should I touch someone I don't know?"

My answer was, "Yes. That's the way you'll get to know the person." Touch needs no introduction.

Of course you will use discretion and sensitivity, but don't forget to reach out to those who are suffering. Your touch will minister greatly to their needs.

Giving AND Receiving

These days it is popular to live independently of others. We mask our independence behind the explanation that we are givers, but a real look into our hearts reveals that giving without receiving is merely another way to maintain control.

When we minister with the goal of relationship—of both giving and receiving—we find that the energy flows out of us and right back in again. If we'll allow the exchange, each life that we touch will, in turn, enrich our world. The ebb and flow is a natural one.

I have a friend who ministers to a large congregation in Southern California. He is always on the go, trying to meet the needs of the people in his church, and I wondered, in the early days of our friendship, how he managed to maintain the energy.

One day, we went together to see a young woman who

had just been diagnosed with terminal cancer. He told me a little bit about her situation as we drove to the hospital, and we prepared our hearts for the familiar conversation.

The visit was a painful one. She was suffering so, and all we could do was hold her and pray for her and share in her grief. By the time we left the hospital room, both of us were close to tears.

I will never forget the attitude of my friend that day. He talked about all that he had learned, in that hour, from me and from the young woman. He had listened intently to what I had shared with her, and he was already trying to put the learning into practice in his life. It was then that I knew the secret of his ability to carry on.

He was not trying to "make it on his own." He took no pride in having all the answers or in offering the "best" comfort. He did not need any credit, nor did he try to maintain a safe distance from the suffering.

My friend understands the simple importance of giving and receiving in the relationships of life. He sees those who are hurting as people who have much to teach him. He is by their side as pastor, true; but he is also by their side to learn. I have marveled at his humility, and at the ease he conveys to those who are in his care. He lets those who are suffering see what they have to offer him as well as what he can offer them. That makes the sufferer's burden so much lighter.

No Need to Be a Hero

In light of the above, we need to remember that heroism should have no place in ministry. You won't get any prizes for meeting everyone's needs alone. In fact, when we fiercely hold on to our precious independence, we violate the basic principles of the body of Christ.

Train other people in your church to help carry the load. Teach those with gifts of compassion and mercy to see God, and then send them out to give that good Gift away. I know that most people want the minister there in

times of sorrow. And I know you want to be there to help
them in their need. You cannot, however, do all of the
mercy-giving alone. There are people in your congregation
who are not only willing to help, but they are gifted of
God to provide strength or mercy in times of need. Train
those people, love them, and use them in service. It will
increase your strength and your ability to minister to the
needs of your sheep.

Truths to Convey

While there are many truths we can convey to those who
are hurting, I have in mind conveying the truths about
God — truths that are often taken for granted until we need
them for our very survival. Let me tell you about those
truths I have needed the most and have learned the most
about in my walk with pain.

A Mirror Image of God

> I know that You can do all things; no plan of
> Yours can be thwarted. . . . Surely I spoke of
> things I did not understand, things too wonder-
> ful for me to know. . . . My ears had heard of You
> but now my eyes have seen You (Job 42:2, 3, 5).

To show someone an accurate picture of God is a tall
order, but in reality, it is exactly what the sufferer needs.
Faced with intense pain, we all hunger to see God — to
know that He is there, that He cares, that He knows what
He is doing, and that He will not let us fall.

You've been amazed as I have, I'm sure, at the number
of people who seem to be void of spiritual awareness
when they need it most. The same people who've been in
church for years and have taught Sunday School can, in
the face of pain, forget everything they've been taught.
Even pastors are not exempt from this scenario.

The single most important task for the minister is to

offer his sheep a true picture of God — a mirror image of the One whose strength sustains, whose love endures, and whose purpose exceeds the boundaries of time.

Make sure you know God. Those who are suffering will be watching to see if you can find any purpose in the pain. They'll be listening to hear if your voice cracks under the weight of insecurity. They'll be waiting to receive the Truth that cannot be silenced by any tragedy or loss.

The way you see God directly influences the way that the sufferers to whom you minister will see God. Make sure you give the picture you want them to believe — the picture that's painted on the scrolls of eternity.

The God of All Comfort

> Praise be to the God and Father of our Lord Jesus Christ, the Father of compassion and the God of all comfort, who comforts us in all our troubles, so that we can comfort those in any trouble with the comfort we ourselves have received from God. For just as the sufferings of Christ flow over into our lives, so also through Christ our comfort overflows. If we are distressed, it is for your comfort and salvation; if we are comforted, it is for your comfort, which produces in you patient endurance of the same sufferings we suffer. And our hope for you is firm, because we know that just as you share in our sufferings, so also you share in our comfort (2 Cor. 1:3-7).

While I certainly don't want to insult you or give you cause for defense, I do want to say that I've seen many a minister try to offer comfort while being only vaguely acquainted with the Comforter Himself. The way you relate to God directly influences the way you give comfort.

The years spent in seminary, preparing for the ministry, are rarely years in which we come face to face with the God of all comfort. We learn much about theology, doctrine, and exegesis; but rarely do we learn about comfort until we are face to face with suffering. The kind of comfort we offer is directly related to the way we've allowed God to comfort us.

You will do yourself a great service if you will sit and do some writing on your own. Write about what you think you would feel and need if you were the recipient of dreadful news or the subject of severe pain and loss. Although such writing won't prepare you for every situation, having thought about your own feelings and needs will help you greatly as you are called upon to minister.

I will never forget seeing a pastor/friend of mine awkwardly standing in the corner of the room after one of his parishioners had lost a child to sudden death. He looked miserable in that corner, and I knew why. He felt helpless to give his parishioners any real comfort, for he had no answers himself—no suggestions, no explanations, no neat conclusions for the message.

All the family needed that day was the comfort that God can give through those who know Him. They needed my friend just to be there and share and pray and cry, but he had rarely allowed himself that privilege.

For the minister to comfort, he must know the God of all comfort. He must be vulnerable, a bit "out of control," and he must be open to the raw pain of loss. Know the God of all comfort so that you can be a conduit of that comfort for those who suffer.

The God Who Is There

> I wait for the Lord, my soul waits, and in His Word I put my hope. My soul waits for the Lord more than watchmen wait for the morning, more than watchmen wait for the morning (Ps. 130:5-6).

In the midst of suffering, some people find it difficult to see God. They search, they hunger, but they are afraid.

You are the physical embodiment of the hope of the believer, and so you become a great light in a darkened room. You remind the one who suffers that God is there.

Think with me, for a moment, about the presence of God in the furnace with Shadrach, Meshach, and Abednego. God was there! And yet, to the eye of the beholder, the furnace had never been hotter.

> Then King Nebuchadnezzar leaped to his feet in amazement and asked his advisors "Weren't there three men that we tied up and threw into the fire?"
>
> They replied, "Certainly, O King."
>
> He said, "Look! I see four men walking around in the fire, unbound and unharmed, and the fourth looks like a son of the gods" (Dan. 3:24-25).

God was there to rescue and comfort the three men whose sights were set on pleasing Him. Even if He had not physically been in the furnace, He still would have been with them. God never leaves His people.

My body is wasting away, as is the case with each of us; but God dwells in the inner man. That inner man is able to grow so beautifully from death and loss and suffering. Paul understood that truth as he wrote his letters to the Corinthian Church (2 Cor. 4:16-17).

We place too much emphasis today on the outer things—the body, riches, achievements—and those things pass away. The dying person has a chance to experience the renewal of the inner man—and that is quite an experience.

Help those who suffer learn that God is with them in the furnace. As the minister of Truth, you can help people encounter the miracle of God's presence.

As a result of my bout with cancer, God has become all

to me, and my understanding of Him has grown and matured and changed and become what I'd always hoped it could be. Suffering has taught me great truths — truths I would not now trade for anything.

I do not feel abandoned in my suffering or left out of God's plan. Nor do I feel as if the suffering is a mistake or as if God's glory will only be revealed some day in the future when my pain is gone. Instead, I feel His glory in me today, in the midst of my suffering, because someone long ago was brave enough to help me discover God and His goodness in the midst of my pain and loss. That discovery, for me, has been the most wonderful part of what could have been some very empty years.

Remember, it will take time for any sufferer to make such a discovery. After all, this world teaches the opposite message. But trust me, God is not glorified only when the suffering is gone. He is, instead, Glory itself. And His glory does not vary in intensity with circumstances. If we will learn to look for Him, He is there.

Face-to-Face

As I read back over my words, I guess what I am really suggesting here is that you spend some time discovering for yourself the true God — the God of all comfort and compassion, justice, and holiness.

When I hear what some ministers preach or see how they live, I wonder why they are so afraid to come face-to-face with truth. It takes a courageous person to choose the truth of Scripture over the popular messages of this world. Be courageous.

We are children of a Father who is big enough to incorporate suffering into His plan. Yet it seems that somewhere in our cultural Christianity we have lost sight of this God that the Bible so clearly and beautifully unfolds. The world and all of the media teach that we are down or unfortunate when we suffer. The opposite is true.

It is in suffering that we come to see Him face-to-face (Job 42:1-5). And it is in suffering that somehow our faith is transformed into perseverance; and perseverance, into character; and character, into hope (Rom. 5:1-5). The result? A hope that does not disappoint. I can't think of a more eternal achievement.

I pray that these thoughts will in some way minister to you, and that they will help you fill your cup to overflowing. We need you, you know, those of us who must look beyond the offerings of this world to the life that is truly life.

May God bless you in your work—and may you know that your labor is not in vain.

Questions to Consider

1. What do you find most difficult about ministering to a dying person or someone in pain?
2. What do you find most difficult about ministering to the family of someone who is suffering or dying?
3. How do you think you would feel if your own life suddenly filled with pain? What do you think you would need from your family? From your minister? From your friends?
4. Make a list of those people in your church who have the gift of compassion and mercy. Commit to train those people so that they can help you fill the needs in your congregation.
5. How did Jesus comfort people in their pain? How has God comforted you in your times of need? Be specific.

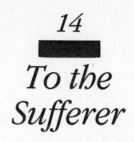

14

To the Sufferer

"In His marvelous and mysterious way, God keeps shaping us until He can see Himself in our lives. The process is long, arduous, complex, and certainly not painless, but it's worth it. And we need not wait to celebrate. We can, if we choose, genuinely celebrate the process." [1]

—Tim Hansel

A Personal Note

All the things I have tried to say in this book are meant to make your life—and mine—a little more meaningful in this world. I wish I could see you, talk with you, and listen to you.

We have all experienced different kinds of pain, but there is a kindred spirit which ties all sufferers together. We have all faced things and died to things which few spectators of suffering can understand. I have tried to reveal some of the process, but it's impossible to give witness to it all.

You have been reading my story, but remember that your story will also be told through the lives and words of your families and friends. Do not suppose that you are insignificant. You are God's child, and your life influences many.

The following reminders may seem obvious to you, particularly if your journey has been like mine, but I want to write them one more time for your sake and for my own sake.

Understand the Importance of Your Journey

First, please believe that whatever is happening to you has significance, both now and in eternity. You may not care too much about eternity right now—particularly if you are suffering under the weight of illness, emotional pain, or financial stress. But the eternal is the only thing that is real.

We live in a culture and time in which we are taught to believe that life will work out "OK" and, perhaps "great" if we make good choices and decisions. I believe that life does work out right, but perhaps not today, not in our time, not now. For now we may have to suffer grief in all kinds of trials (1 Peter 1:6-7), but those trials are not empty of meaning.

I often read about Job or Jeremiah or Paul as I seek to come to grips with the ever-present reality of physical pain. What I learn from these three men is simple. If this world were the end, in and of itself, then what we believe would be worth nothing. But if God really is who He claims to be, and if eternity is indeed the culmination of this life, then the truths of Scripture are worth everything we endure in this life—even the losses.

Perhaps you have children you must leave behind or maybe you've lost someone you love or maybe your body or heart is racked with pain, and you find little comfort in spiritual battles or purposes. I understand. But the spiritual realm is real, and understanding that makes all the difference in this world.

I think we sufferers are fortunate, not because we enjoy pain, but because pain has a way of making the immaterial disappear in the search for what is true. Because we can turn nowhere else for relief, we turn to God and begin to discern what life and death and sacrifice and compassion are really all about.

Hold on to the eternal. It is not an empty hope or an excuse, as some would accuse. The eternal perspective of God and this life is like the foundation of a house. Though we spend our time decorating walls and buying furniture to go in that house, the foundation is the ground upon which we stand. When the storm comes, only a strong foundation matters. The frills hold little significance in the real tests of life.

Open up your heart to the journey. God is always there, though we cannot always see Him. And He loves us much more than we can now understand. When the pain is too much to bear, hand some of it to Jesus. I literally picture Him picking up the load as I walk with Him and tell Him of my struggles. The sufferings of this world will be over soon, yet the lessons we learn from them will have eternal significance.

Be Honest with Loved Ones

Second, let me encourage you to be honest with your family members and friends about what you need. I have spent many a lonely day wishing my loved ones understood what I have neglected to tell them.

Those who love you are caught in the suffering as much as you are, and perhaps even more. They feel helpless to do anything to relieve the pain, and so they flounder through this strange event that they never dreamed would happen to you—or to them.

They need you to tell them what is going on inside of you and what you need from them. You are the sufferer, and they need to take their cues from you.

Accept Responsibility

I imagine you are fed up with lectures about responsibility, but I know of no more important lesson for the person in pain. No one else can accept our load, even though we may feel that load is too heavy to bear.

God promises that nothing He gives is too cumbersome, and we must keep in mind that He has reason to allow suffering in our lives.

Observers of pain seem to want to jump right in to try their hand at making it all OK. Accept the help—burdens *are* meant to be shared. But hold on to the fact that this is your pain, and you are the one equipped to deal with that pain.

We all need one another, but we also need to carry our own load. There are times when it's appropriate to release your pain to another's care, but generally, you must bear the spiritual and emotional responsibility for your pain. God has much in store for those of us who suffer, and it's important that we take hold of maturity.

Be Honest with Your Doctor

This suggestion is easier said than done, but it is an important part of the process. Don't be afraid to tell your doctor what you want. Very simply, it is your body and your life. Even though physicians are trained in the care and treatment of the body, they are not trained in the art of knowing you.

I am a people-pleaser, so much of my early bout with cancer was spent trying to please doctors as well as family members and friends. I have had to learn to tell others what I want, even if they disagree.

Doctors are taught to do all they can to make our physical condition better. It is difficult for them to turn loose and let us control our own decisions. Be brave and be honest. You will feel better about you if *you* are the one making the decisions for your own care.

Accept the Gift of Love

Fourth, please don't feel bad about letting other people see your weaknesses or minister to you in your need. We are raised to be self-sufficient, but the truth is, we really do need each other.

I have known mothers with cancer who refuse to see their children once the disease is apparent. I have watched men suffer and refuse to allow their wives or their children to care for their basic needs. I have watched families turn away friends because they hate to ask for help. And I have seen financial support rejected on the grounds that we shouldn't take from other people.

When your children were young, did you begrudge them care? If your own friend were dying, wouldn't you want to help?

We really do need one another. And if we can't let someone step in and love us once the pretty exterior is gone, what is friendship all about? It is a joy to serve someone who is suffering. Please don't deprive people of that joy.

Look for Purpose

Lastly, look for purpose today and every day. It is there, but it takes some discovery to begin to see our value in terms of *being* rather than *doing*.

I stayed with a woman one day who was no longer able to do anything for her family. She was confined to a hospital bed in the living room, and she cried because she could no longer cook or clean or serve in the ways that had characterized her life for years.

If you are too ill to get out of bed, then be creative. Write notes of encouragement or share your thoughts with your family and friends on a tape recorder. Have your minister bring you a list of the prayer requests from the church. Just think of the good you can do as you pray for people in their need. Tell your family and friends what you are learning. Someday, they may need to know the very same lessons, and hearing from you today will greatly help them in their own suffering tomorrow. We forget that no one knows how to suffer, so we need all the help we can get. The point is, even in your pain, you can be a real encouragement to others. Your life is not without purpose.

You are useful—it just isn't fleshed out in the ways that it used to be. Don't let the suffering mask who you are; you are the same beloved friend, daughter, son, mother, father, or spouse that you've always been.

If you are at the beginning of your suffering, it will take time for the words in this book to speak to you. We who suffer are in shock, at first, and then we struggle with accepting the reality of our situation. We do have a choice in how we respond. We can either live angrily and refuse to see good, or we can accept the reality of suffering's presence and choose to see God in its midst.

Wherever you are in the process, I encourage you to choose God. His ways have never led to darkness, they have never been more than we can bear, they have never been fruitless, and they have never been without purpose. I know the struggles: weariness, lack of energy, depression, anger, discouragement, frustration. But I also know the joys: loving and receiving love, feeling God's strength when yours is gone, understanding Scripture in a whole new way, holding each day—each moment—as significant, growing and maturing in ways you'd never dreamed.

> Three times I pleaded with the Lord to take [the thorn in the flesh] away from me. But He said to me, "My grace is sufficient for you, for My power is made perfect in weakness." Therefore, I will boast all the more gladly about my weaknesses, so that Christ's power may rest on me. That is

why, for Christ's sake, I delight in weaknesses, in
insults, in hardships, in persecutions, in difficulties. For when I am weak, then I am strong
(2 Cor. 12:8-10).

I send my love and my prayers to you in your suffering
and ask you to keep your eyes upon God. He is there, and
He will never leave you: "In this world you will have trouble. But take heart! I have overcome the world" (John
16:33).

Questions to Consider

1. With what do you struggle most in your suffering?
2. Whom do you really trust to understand what you're
   going through and to be there for you? If there is no
   one, find someone. People do care.
3. What are some of the things you've learned from your
   frailty? From your need for God? From your friends and
   family?
4. What do you find hardest to accept about your frailty?
   What do you think God can teach you from this particular difficulty?
5. Write a letter (or if you're unable to write, talk into a
   tape recorder) to each of the key people in your life.
   Tell those people what you are feeling, what you need
   from them, and what you want them to understand.

15

To the Physician

"I knew more than I could ever use. I saw more than I could ever prevent. But nothing I knew nor anything I saw was ever as miraculous as a soul coming to God. Though I lived as a physician, I died in the hands of the mender of souls. How I wish I had known what was really important in the years of my youth." [1]

—A French physician

Letter from a Patient

Perhaps it is presumptuous of me to write to men and women who are so specifically trained. Certainly, I cannot presume to know the myriad of things you know about the human body, diseases, medicine, etc., but I would like to tell you a few things that have been important to me in my battle with cancer.

I have shared these thoughts with physicians and medical students throughout the United States and in countries overseas. They are simple thoughts, but they warrant discussion. When a person is suffering, the simple is significant.

Unique Patients

> For You created my inmost being; You knit me together in my mother's womb. I praise You because I am fearfully and wonderfully made; Your works are wonderful, I know that full well (Ps. 139:13-14).

The patient who comes to you is as individual as the stars in the sky. A physician sees the same things day in and day out: cancer, disease, depression, pain, death. You may know the illness, but you don't know the person.

I say this simply to remind you that what may be commonplace to you is brand-new to your patient. Though the disease may be a conventional one, the person inside that troubled body is a unique creation of God. Both the body and the individual need your support.

A Physician's Limitations

A physician's hands are skillful hands. They can offer relief and the best care available, but they do not possess the power to heal. Only God can heal. It is important for you to help the patient accept that reality. Please don't lose sight of your limitations—they are there for a reason.

Inside every hurting body is a person who knows you do not hold the keys to life and death, but we want to think you hold those keys so that we can feel more secure. The shock of a newly discovered illness can be severe.

Be gentle, but please don't feel as if you need to make promises you cannot keep. It is important that the patient and the family carry their portion of the load.

Live With God's Perspective

There is much within a physician's grasp to lessen the burden of the sufferer. Indeed, God has given you a great responsibility, but it is not to be God. While we want you to do what is wise, try not to place what you know to be true about medicine ahead of what you know to be true about God and Christianity. Be committed, first, to Truth.

Be a care-giver who uses your abilities to provide the best possible support for a patient, but make sure that you wisely consider just what that support ought to be. Tune in to both the individual and to God. The combination is essential.

I have watched doctors do everything they can to keep a body alive a few more days. I have watched doctors seem almost obsessed with trying one more drug or treatment. An observer of such scenarios would say that the doctor must see death as failure or physical days in this world as the greater gain.

Death is not failure, neither is suffering a mistake. God is in control. And when a believer goes home, that believer faces the most wonderful life you and I can now imagine.

I am not suggesting that you provide your patients with poor care or that you stand by and watch whenever a patient is dying. I am merely saying: hold on to what you believe about God. Live with God's perspectives—try to see things His way; and share with your patients the truths that form your whole approach to life.

Quality Time, Not Quantity

Involvement is the glue that holds life together. We are all involved in one another's lives, whether we like it or not. As a physician, you *do* have an impact on the personal lives of those who come to you for care. It is up to you just what impact that will be.

I am not asking you to spend hours counseling your patients in the finer arts of spirituality. I know that your time is limited. I am not asking you to take each patient on as a project. I am asking you to live out your faith and to treat the patient, while in your care, with the kind of love and concern you receive from God. It is a myth that loving takes more time than not getting involved.

A smile, a touch, a prayer, a word of encouragement, a life of faith, a personal example of God's grace can all be part of the routine exam. Please take time to love—spend quality time with those who seek your support.

Honesty

Finally, the last thing I am asking of you is honesty. Patients need to know what is going on in their lives. They need to hear the truth about their situations so that they can adjust and grow and find strength to face whatever the problem may be.

As a patient, I want to know what is wrong with me, how you see my condition, what you think will happen, and what you think I should do. I want to know so that I can prepare, and so that life, however long, short, or painful, might be lived to the best of my ability.

When I was a child, I was afraid of the dark. My parents solved the fear by letting me sleep with lights on, and it worked—for a time. The problem came when I went away to college and my roommate wasn't too keen on sleeping with all the lights left on!

Had my parents turned out the lights when I was a child and sat by my bed for a night or two, I would have worked through the problem. I might have cried and felt afraid, but several weeks of sleeping in the dark would have taught me that I had no reason to be afraid.

A patient might weep, feel afraid, become depressed, or unleash anger when told the truth about the situation, but the truth will eventually set that person free to live appropriately with the situation. It just takes honesty and time. Learn to help both family and patient deal with the reality—in relationship to you, and in relationship to one another.

Please know that you are very much appreciated—

just for your presence and your commitment. The pressure of such a job is immense, I know, but the service you offer is an eternal gift. Thank you, on behalf of all who will live and die in your care. May God bless you in your work.

Questions to Consider

1. What have been your most difficult realizations in your practice as a physician?
2. How has your faith in God changed and grown?
3. How have you incorporated your faith into your service? Can you see other ways in which you might do this?
4. How do you view death? Is it difficult to grasp God's perspective when you are trained in the art of mending?
5. Think back over some of your most memorable patients. What has made those patients stand out in your mind? What insights have you gained from them?

Epilogue

It's All in How You Choose to See

Safe Within the Shadow

Suffering to maturity, dying to live, and losing to find are all seeming paradoxes of a world we only begin to comprehend. But God assures us of His truth and of the hope that is ours for all eternity.

I am still living in pain at the writing of this book. And I am still learning more and more about God in the midst of my suffering. I will forever be grateful to my family and my friends who have stayed by my side in the struggle.

I have learned to live daily with the suffering and to take one step at a time. It's funny, but I feel most afraid when I try to imagine living this way for the next ten or twenty years. In those moments, I remind myself that the strength will be there as I need it—not before.

Whether my days are one or ten thousand, I know I will witness the working out of God's grace in my life. He has a plan, and I am a vital part of that plan.

I am thankful to be where I am and where I've been. If God chooses to lift the suffering, I will rejoice, but it is no longer necessary. More than anything, I want to continue to live with the same hunger and intensity that He's placed within me these past years. I want to live serving Him and pleasing Him and thirsting after His Truths.

I want to love others and share in their journeys, passing on insights which have become a part of me. I want to experience what God thinks I need and to trust His judgment. I never want to lose sight of who God is or who I am in His wonderful scheme. And I want the deaths I have died always to remind me of life.

God is good, and He gives good gifts to His children. God works good in our lives, and He intends His good to emerge from even the most difficult of circumstances. I believe this is true, and I have seen Him work. We have nothing to fear.

My prayer is the same as Paul's. It is the prayer I pray as I struggle along, and it is the prayer I pray for everyone else on this world's pilgrimage:

> I want to know Christ and the power of His resurrection and the fellowship of sharing in His sufferings, becoming like Him in His death, and so, somehow, to attain to the resurrection from the dead (Phil. 3:10).

Maturity is a process, and this world's sufferings have their place. Allow God to use them to mold you into His very image. After all, we are clay in the Potter's hand, and we are safe—within the shadow.

Notes

CHAPTER 1: Beginning Thoughts
1. John Claypool, *Tracks of a Fellow Struggler* (Waco: Word Books, 1974), pp. 13, 15.

CHAPTER 2: I Heard the Steeple Chiming
1. Paul Brandt and Philip Yancey, *Fearfully and Wonderfully Made* (Grand Rapids: Zondervan, 1980), p. 59.

CHAPTER 3: A Single Seed
1. C.S. Lewis, *Chronicles of Narnia* (New York: Macmillan Publishing Co., 1950).

CHAPTER 4: Through the Eye of a Needle
1. John Bunyan, *The Pilgrim's Progress* (Massachusetts: Paraclete Press, 1982), p. 79.

CHAPTER 5: Hello, World
1. Edith Schaeffer, *The Art of Life* (Westchester, Ill: Crossway Books, 1987), p. 125.

CHAPTER 6: Welcome Home, Uncle Sam
1. Charles Swindoll, *Dropping Your Guard* (Waco: Word Books, 1983), p. 192.
2. Mote and Bradbury, "The Solid Rock"

CHAPTER 7: Hard Days for Love
1. Marilee Dunker, *A Braver Song to Sing* (Grand Rapids: Zondervan, 1987), p. 42.

CHAPTER 8: Pain as Companion
1. Amy Carmichael, "Nothing in the House" (Fort Washington, Pa.: Christian Literature Crusade).

CHAPTER 9: Clay in the Potter's Hand
1. Tim Hansel, *Choosing Joy* (Elgin, Ill.: David C. Cook Publishing, 1985), pp. 122-123.

CHAPTER 10: Healing from the Inside Out
1. Philip Yancey, *Disappointment with God* (Grand Rapids: Zondervan, 1988), p. '186.
2. Ibid., p. 147.
3. Concerning the benefits in the atonement, the Expositor's Bible Commentary records, "It should be stated that this discussion cannot be used to justify healing on demand. This text (Matthew 8:16-17) and others clearly teach that there is healing in the atonement; but similarly there is the promise of a resurrection body in the atonement, even if believers do not inherit it until the Parousia. From the perspective of the New Testament writers, the Cross is the basis for all the benefits that accrue to believers; but this does not mean that all such benefits can be secured at the present time on demand, any more than we have the right and power to demand our resurrection bodies. Modern Christians should avoid the principle danger of Corinth, viz. an over-realized eschatology which demands blessing that may not be ours till the end of the age." *The Expositor's Bible Commentary,* Frank Gaebelein, editor, Zondervan, 1984, pp. 206-207.
4. Another passage often used to supplement the belief that faith heals is Matthew 18:19. "Again I tell you that if two of you on earth agree about anything you ask for, it will be done for you by My Father in heaven." It should be noted that this passage deals with judging a legal matter or settling a dispute. Though they are often used as such, these verses are not a promise regarding prayer.

CHAPTER 11: The Good Gifts of God
1. Tim Hansel, *Choosing Joy* (Elgin, Ill.: David C. Cook, 1985), p. 117.
2. W.E. Vine, *An Expository Dictionary of New Testament Words* (Old Tappan, N.J.: Fleming H. Revell Company, 1940).
3. Philip Yancey, *Disappointment with God* (Grand Rapids: Zondervan, 1988), p. 67.

CHAPTER 12: To Family and Friends
1. Tim Hansel, *Choosing Joy* (Elgin, Ill.: David C. Cook Publishing, 1985), p. 116.

CHAPTER 13: To the Minister
1. Philip Yancey, *Disappointment with God* (Grand Rapids: Zondervan, 1988), p. 26.

CHAPTER 14: To the Sufferer
1. Tim Hansel, *Choosing Joy* (Elgin, Ill.: David C. Cook, 1985), pp. 142-143.

CHAPTER 15: To the Physician
1. Anonymous notation from a physician in the French Revolution.